the little book of

GOAT YOGA

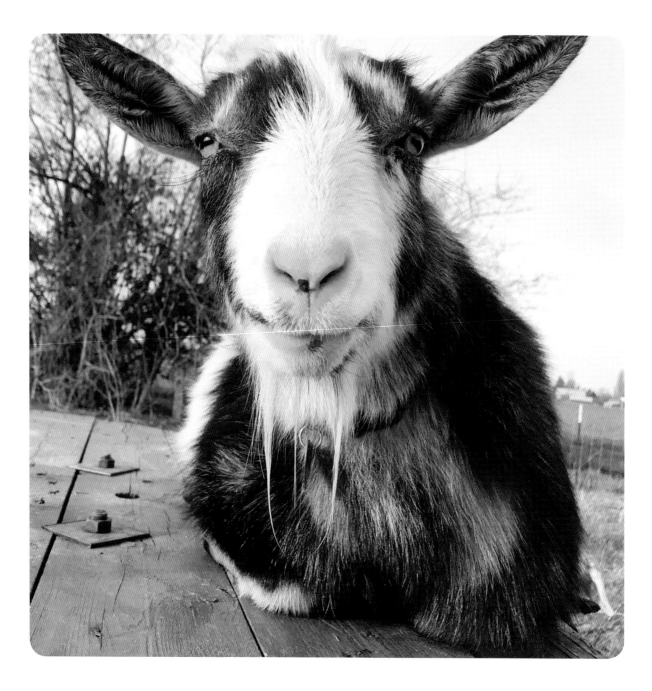

the little book of
GOAT YOGA

POSES & WISDOM
TO INSPIRE YOUR PRACTICE

LAINEY MORSE

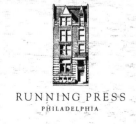

Running Press
PHILADELPHIA

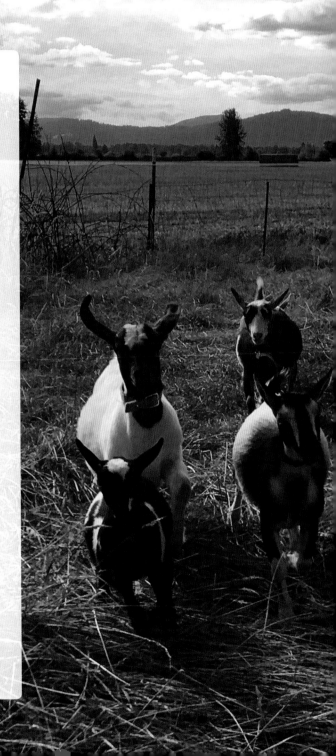

Running Press
Hachette Book Group
1290 Avenue of the Americas, New York, NY 10104
www.runningpress.com
@Running_Press

Printed in China

First Edition: November 2018

Published by Running Press, an imprint of Perseus Books, LLC, a subsidiary of Hachette Book Group, Inc. The Running Press name and logo is a trademark of the Hachette Book Group.

The Hachette Speakers Bureau provides a wide range of authors for speaking events. To find out more, go to www.hachettespeakersbureau.com or call (866) 376-6591.

The publisher is not responsible for websites (or their content) that are not owned by the publisher.

White wood background photo © Gettyimages.com/Antonel; dark wood background photo © Gettyimages.com/Plateresca.

Photographs pages 34, 36, 40, 44, 48, 50, 54, 58, 62, 63, 67, 70–72, 76, 80, 86, 87, 90, 94, 96, 100, 105, 108, 113 by Ashley Marvin; page 1 by Sean Scorvo; page 30 by Kristi McLean; page 56 by Melanie Heistand. All other photographs by Lainey Morse.

Print book cover and interior design by Ashley Todd.

Library of Congress Control Number: 2018938591

ISBNs: 978-0-7624-6528-6 (paperback), 978-0-7624-6526-2 (ebook)

1010

10 9 8 7 6 5 4 3 2 1

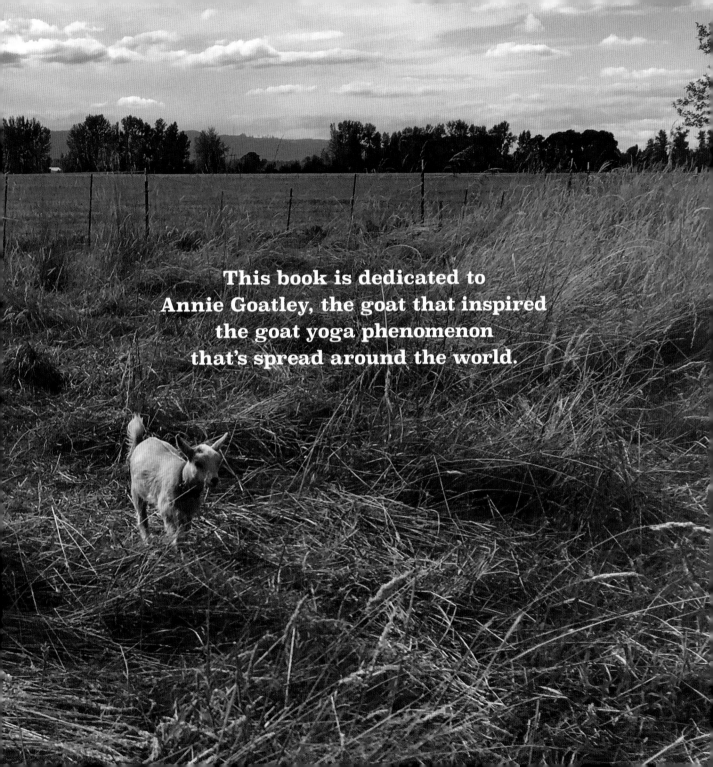

This book is dedicated to
Annie Goatley, the goat that inspired
the goat yoga phenomenon
that's spread around the world.

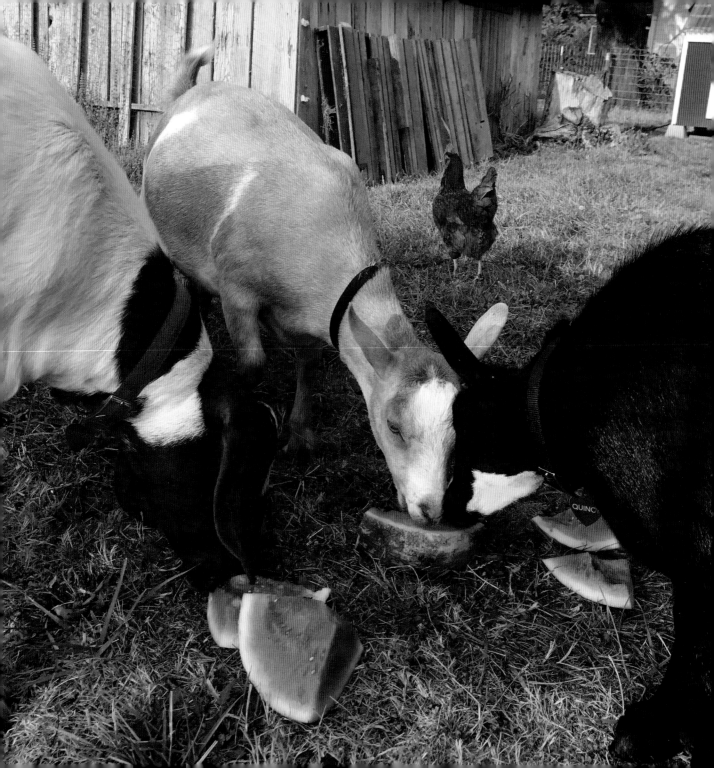

CONTENTS

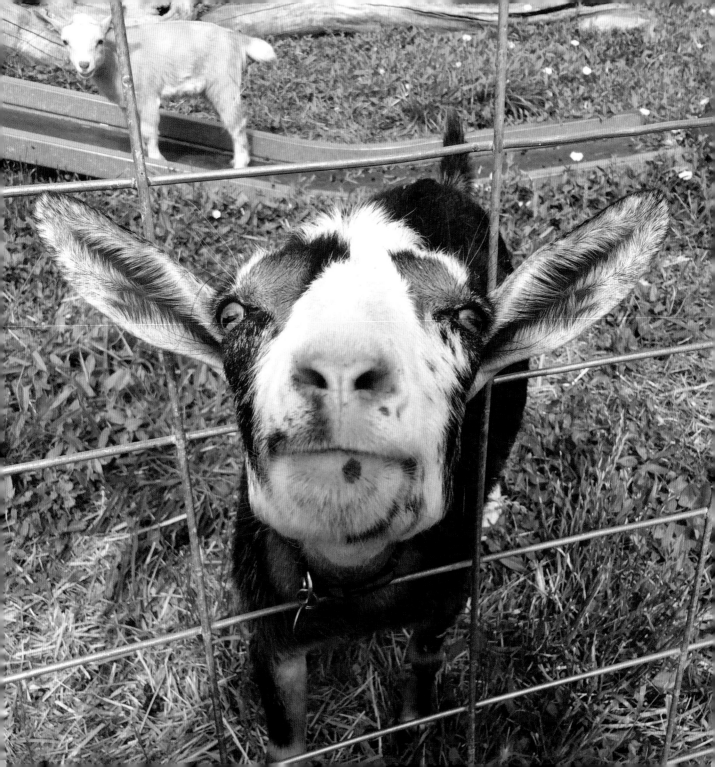

INTRODUCTION

It's a Goat Thing

I've been an animal lover all my life. When I was a child living in Muskegon, Michigan, my family always raised dogs, so I was constantly surrounded by furry four-legged friends. I loved those dogs, but the animals I had always wanted were goats—I just never lived in a spot where I could have them. That all changed once I moved to my farm in Oregon 4 years ago at a point in my life when I was going through many transitions: I had asked my husband of 10 years for a divorce. A few months later, I was diagnosed with an autoimmune disease called Sjögren's syndrome. The only escape from the emotional and physical pain I was experiencing at that time was animal-assisted therapy. That's why the very first thing I did when I settled into my farm (aptly named "No Regrets") was get chickens, barn cats, and my long-awaited goats. I started with two: Ansel and Adams.

I looked forward to coming home from work every day so I could go out in the field or in the barn and spend time with the goats. Goats are incredibly special animals: they possess a very calming demeanor, yet they're also really mischievous and do things that make you laugh all the time.

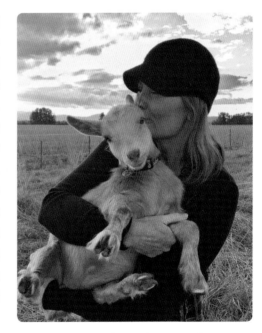

Nuzzling with Annie on my farm.

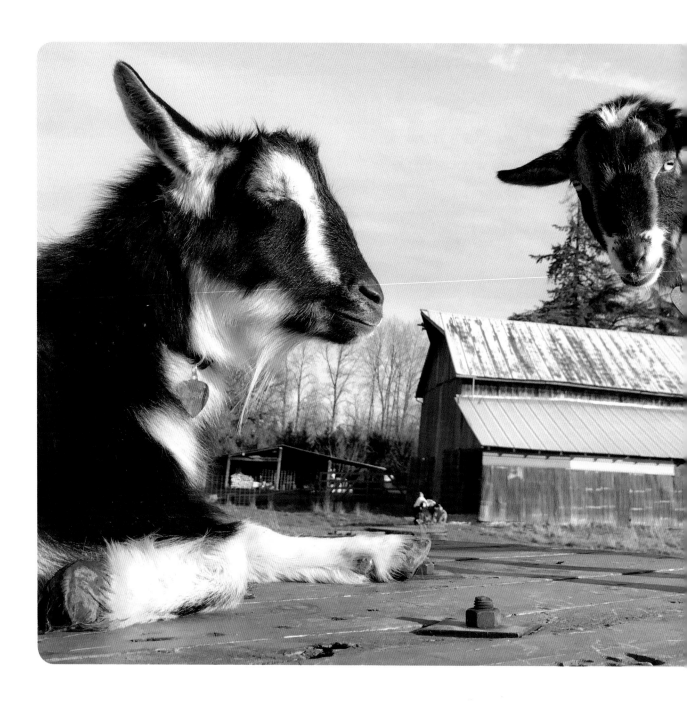

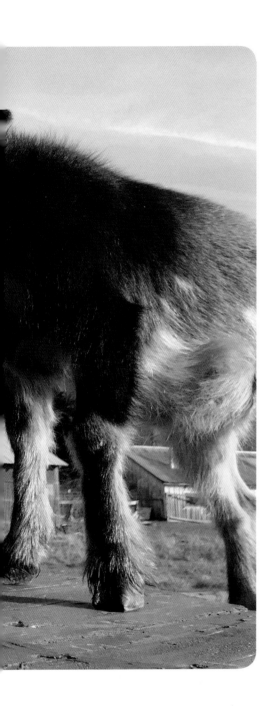

It's the mixture of those two qualities that makes them such unique animals and why I always find time with them to be so therapeutic. They are ruminants that chew their cud (a portion of food that returns from a ruminant's stomach to the mouth to be chewed for the second time) for around 8 hours a day. Cud chewing is a very methodical and meditative process, which, as a human, is very calming and fascinating to watch: you snap into the present moment and don't think of anything else.

Most of the time, I enjoyed my goats by myself, but I gradually started inviting other people over who I knew were stressed out or ill—whether it was just a bad day or something more serious, I could see that being with goats really made people happy. I started hosting weekly gatherings where friends could come and enjoy some drinks, conversation, and animal therapy—I called the nights Goat Happy Hour, and I couldn't believe the response. Attendees enjoyed their wine, sure, but I knew what they really wanted was a good snuggle with one of the goats.

At one of the Goat Happy Hours, Heather Davis, an attendee who happened to be a yoga instructor, and I were standing out in the field surrounded by goats. As she observed the beauty around us, she suggested holding a yoga class at the farm. Though I thought it was a great idea, I warned her that goats would definitely climb all over the humans if they were anywhere near the class. She was not deterred; in fact, that's exactly what she had in mind! We decided to give it a go—since I was a photographer, I had her out to do a promo shoot to see how "yoga with goats" might look and if we could get anyone to come to the farm for such a thing. Sure enough, as soon as Heather got into a pose, my baby goat Annie jumped onto her back. It was such a spontaneous, fun, and happy moment, and with that photo, goat yoga was born.

After seeing the pure joy on Heather's face as Annie accompanied her through her flow, I knew we were on to something. I saw how my Goat Happy Hours brought people joy, so why not pair goats and yoga? The two seemed to fit perfectly together: goats are meditative, calm, peaceful creatures who aren't afraid of a little exercise—who better to accompany yogis through their poses? We held our first class the next week, and 40 people happily showed up.

After hearing about us, a writer at a local publication, *Modern Farmer*, wanted to do a story on our goat yoga classes. I gladly sent the writer pictures of the first class and told him I thought the magazine's readers might think this was fun, but I had no big expectations. Almost immediately, though, the article went viral. After the *Oregonian* saw the *Modern Farmer* piece, they did a feature about goat yoga, and my life changed forever: suddenly, there was a 2,400-person waiting list for the classes, and I was doing 30 to 40 media interviews a day. I started receiving e-mails from people around the world saying how just reading about the classes and seeing pictures of the goats had helped them cope with depression, cancer, chronic illness, daily stress, and more. It seemed something so simple and pure—goats and yoga!—was dramatically changing people's lives. It was at that point that I quit my job of 10 years and decided to

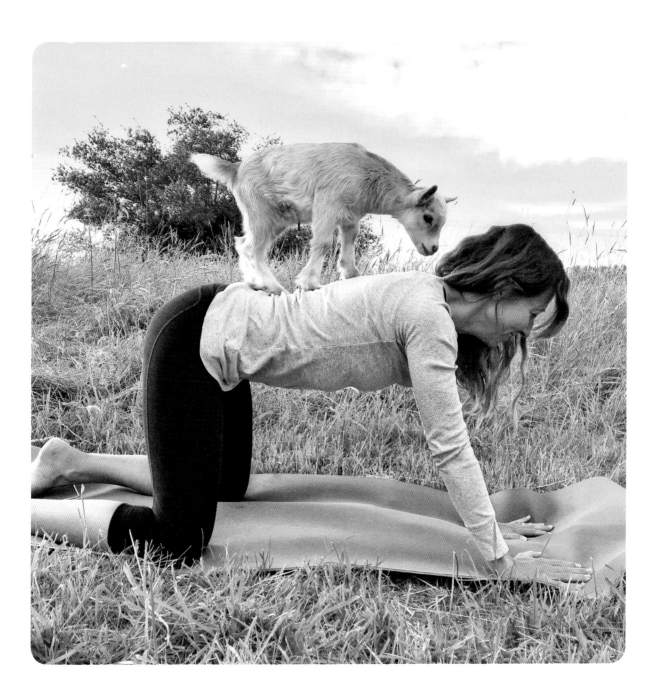

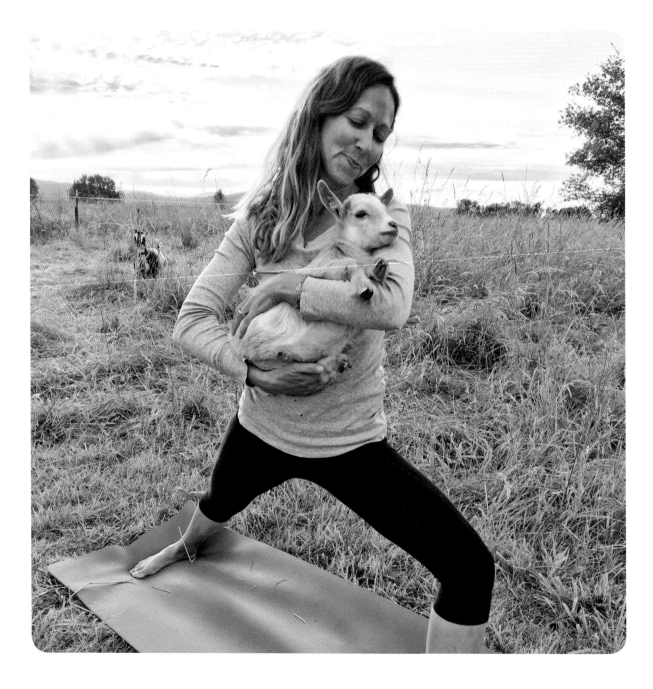

focus solely on the farm, on goat yoga, and on making this my life's work. It's the best decision I ever made!

How to Use This Book

My hope is that *The Little Book of Goat Yoga* will help you take a little piece of "goat namaste" with you wherever you go throughout your day. With adorable photos of my beloved goats throughout and a yoga practice crafted by Heather, this book is like a portable goat yoga class—the next best thing to enjoying a class in person.

WHAT IF I DON'T HAVE A GOAT?

Unfortunately, this book doesn't come with your very own baby goat (I wish!), but don't worry: you can still enjoy a goat yoga practice without a furry friend. For the purposes of this book, all you'll need is a yoga mat, comfortable clothes in which you can move easily, and maybe a yoga block or strap. Allow the "goatations" interspersed throughout the book to keep your practice light and full of joy, just like my goats do for people in person. And if you have a cat, dog, or other curious pet who wants to join you on your mat as you move through the poses, let him! He might interrupt your Chair Pose, but that's the essence of goat yoga: allowing yourself to enjoy the practice however it unfolds.

We've broken this book into three sections:

CONNECT My perspective on life is that it is important to be still occasionally and not take myself too seriously. People today have such busy schedules that they desperately need a way they can connect with themselves and simply enjoy life in the moment. Let's face it, moments of peacefulness and pure bliss are hard to come by. This section will ease you into connecting with yourself by letting go of the stresses you face.

ENGAGE Every yoga practice requires engaging your mind, body, and spirit. Goat yoga is no different. Each pose in this section is designed to engage and strengthen your core. A strong core is just as much physical as it is mental. It's pretty hard to have a weak core with an adorable goat staring at you.

RESTORE Restorative yoga enhances your flexibility, deeply relaxes your body, and stills your mind. In this section, you will learn poses that will boost your immune system, enhance your mood, balance your nervous system, and increase your capacity for compassion toward yourself.

Now let's goat to it! Namaste!

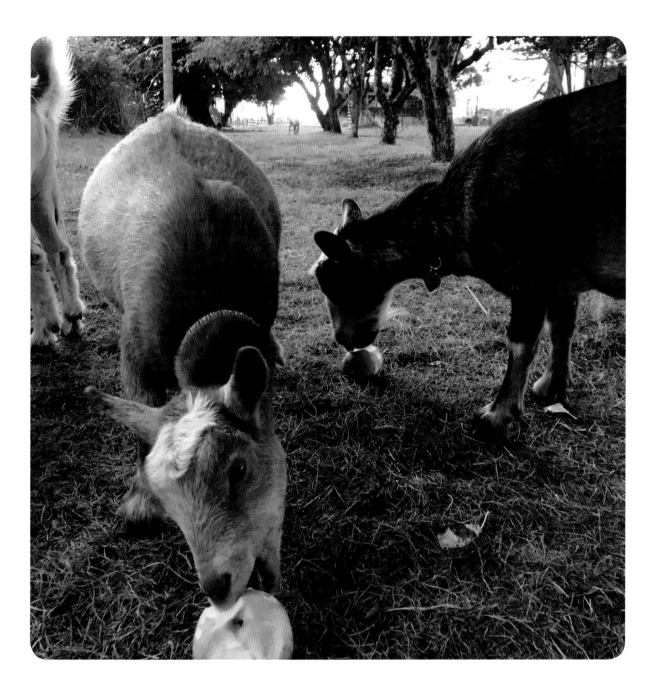

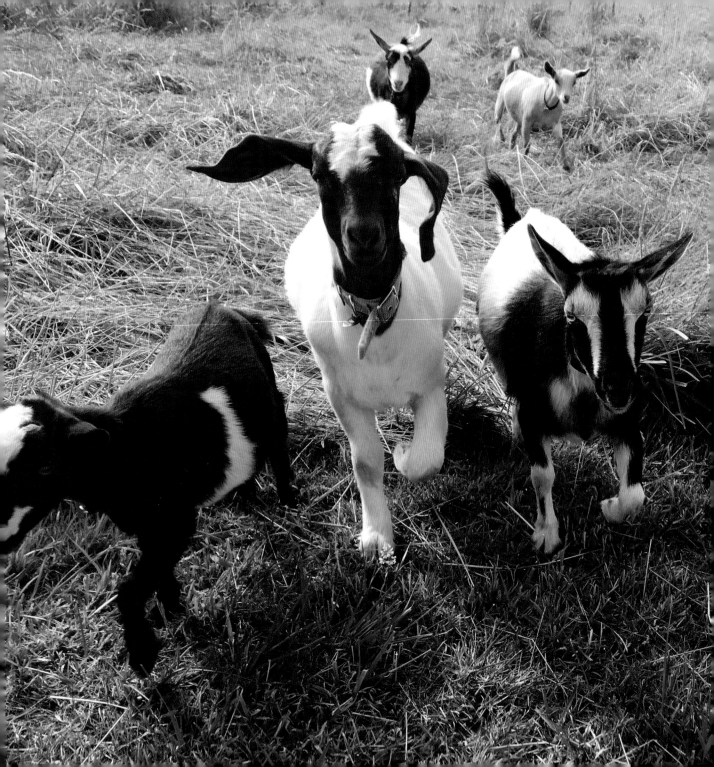

MEET the GOATS

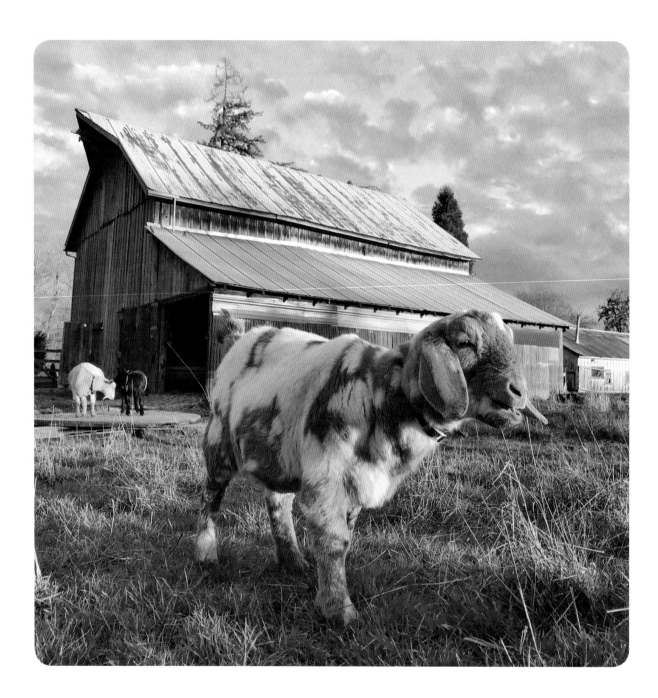

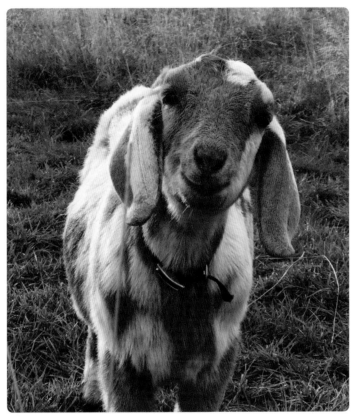

Romeo

My name is Romeo and I am the self-proclaimed ladies' man (goat) on the farm. I melt the hearts of everyone I meet. In fact, I bring them to their knees (for Child's Pose) with my irresistible charm. My floppy ears and dreamy eyes don't hurt, either. I have a heart-shaped patch of white fur on the top of my head, making it the perfect spot for a love pat before yogis strike their next pose. I am also renowned for being very sweet and affectionate . . . oh, and yes, I'm single.

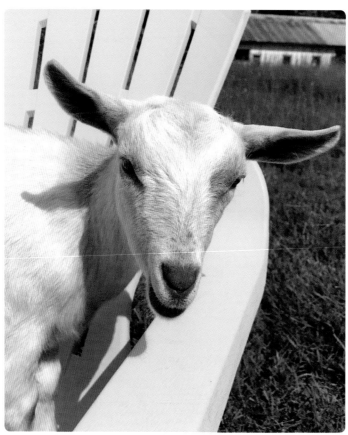

Poppy

My name is Poppy and I have a ton of goattitude! Like a feisty firecracker, I love to jump around, but my favorite place to be is up high, standing on top of anything and everything—especially humans in yoga poses such as the Table Top. Here in goat yoga, I demand excellence! I want to see yogis sweat (so I can take a nap on their backs).

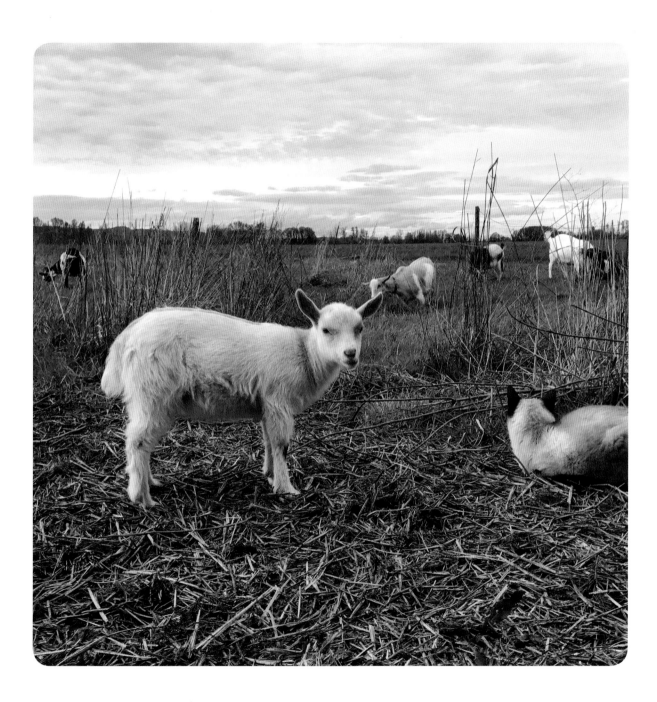

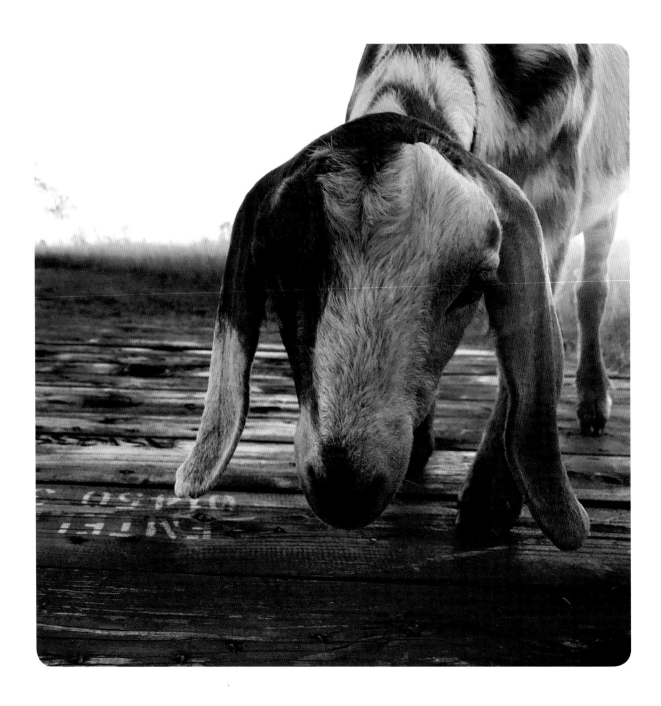

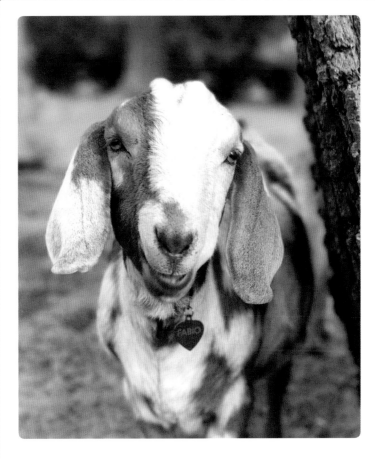

Fabio

I'm often mistaken for that guy who was on the cover of romance novels, but let's be honest: I am way better looking. My presence in class never goes unnoticed, and when I see someone struggling, I just whisper, "You've goat this!" It always works.

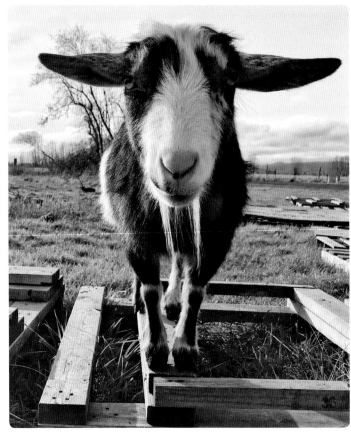

Ansel

The name? Ansel. The profession? Human snuggler. I'm a *goat* listener, so once you have my ear—and if you can manage some words while holding a Plank position—your problems will melt away. I'd say that makes me the GOAT (greatest of all time).

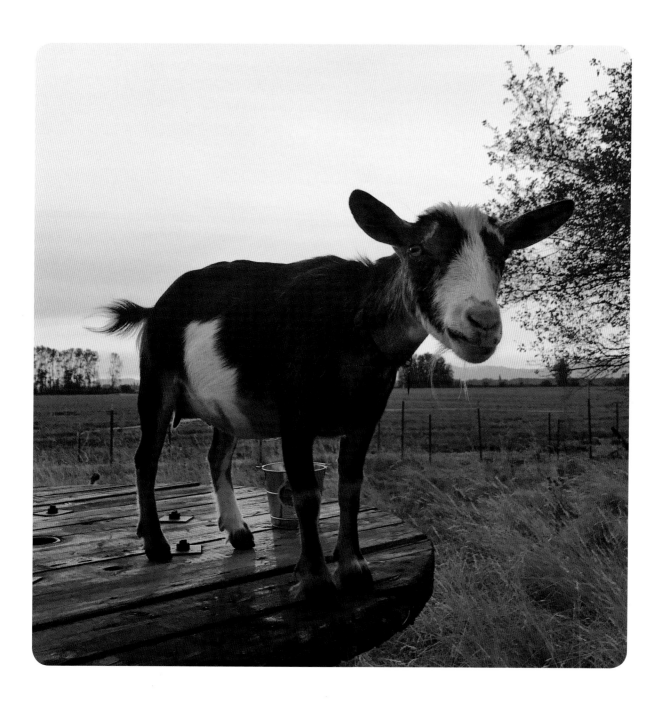

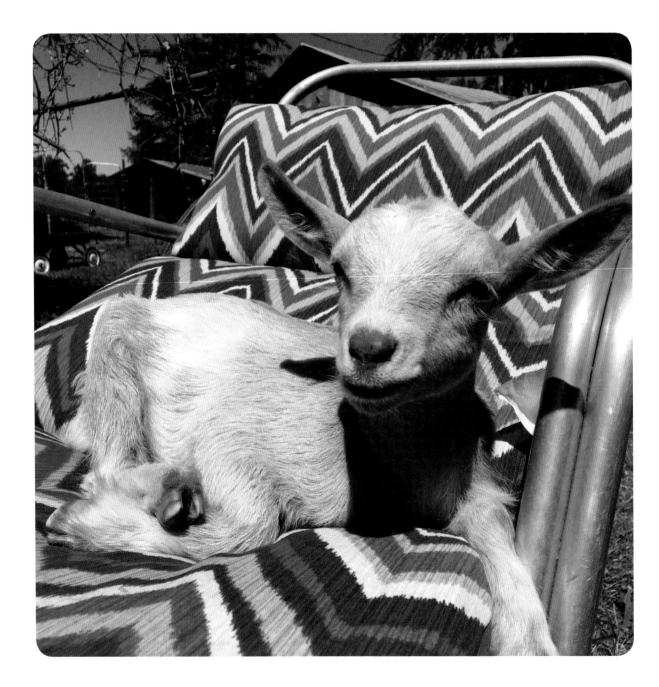

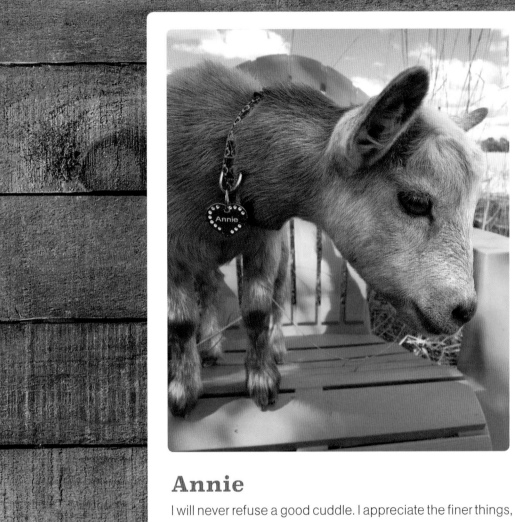

Annie

I will never refuse a good cuddle. I appreciate the finer things, like my bling collar (I'm the goat featured in our logo and I know I'm special), but I also love being around humans. If they're happy, I'm happy. PS: Presents are always welcome!

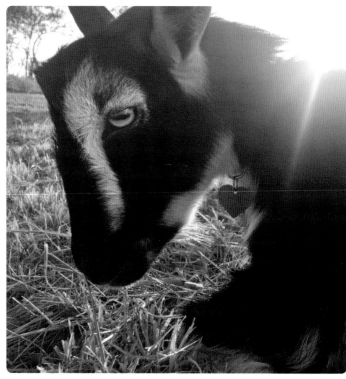

Adams

When I'm not studying US history or working on my thesis, I can be found assisting yogis with Tree Pose. Don't you just love the beginning of my next speech: "Four score and seven goats ago . . ."?

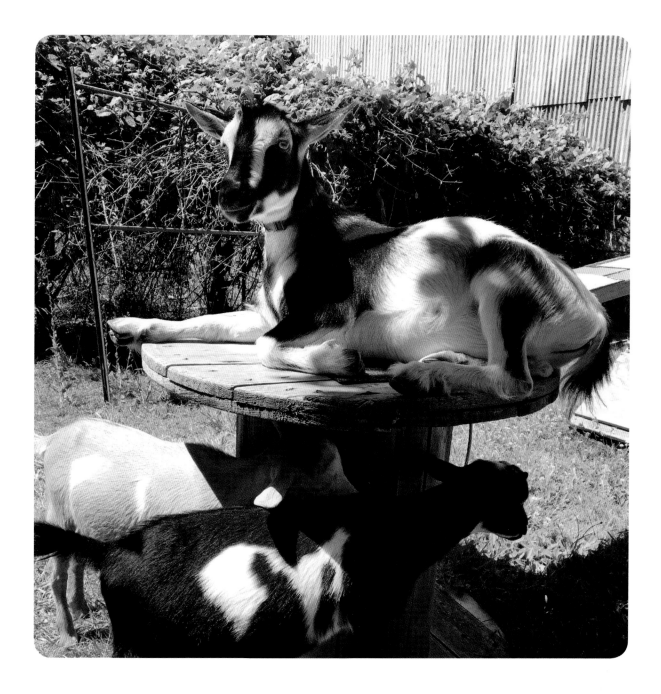

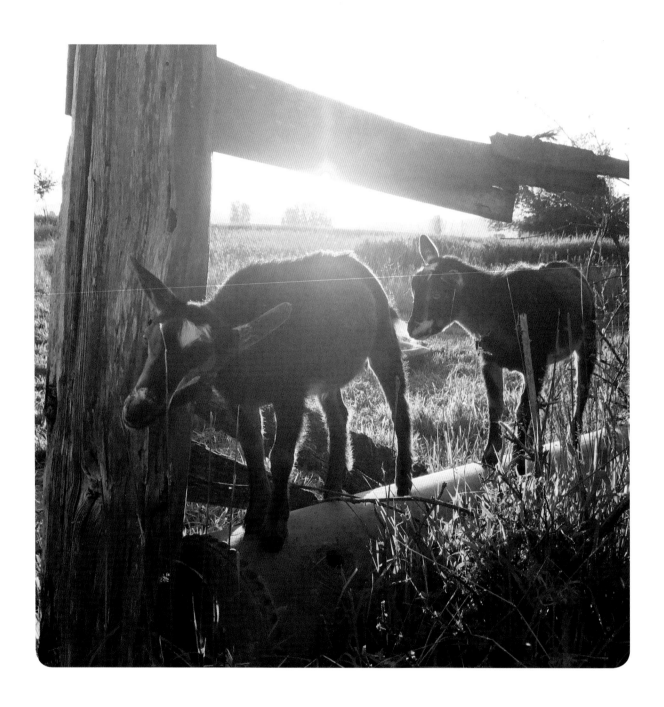

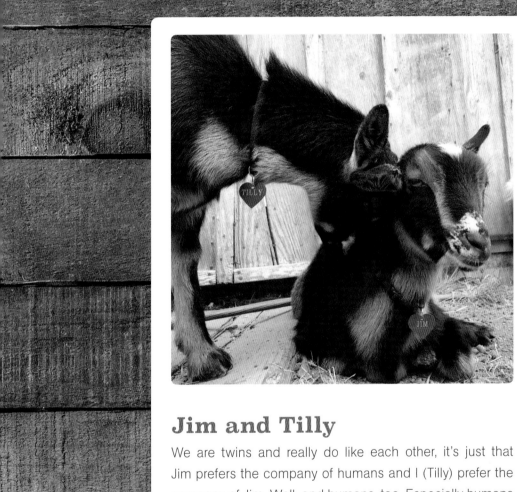

Jim and Tilly

We are twins and really do like each other, it's just that Jim prefers the company of humans and I (Tilly) prefer the company of Jim. Well, and humans, too. Especially humans who do yoga.

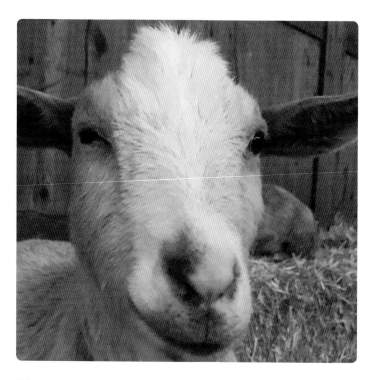

Preston

I love the camera. I really do. I understand that some people would rather do a yoga pose than pose for a picture with me, but sometimes my feelings get hurt.

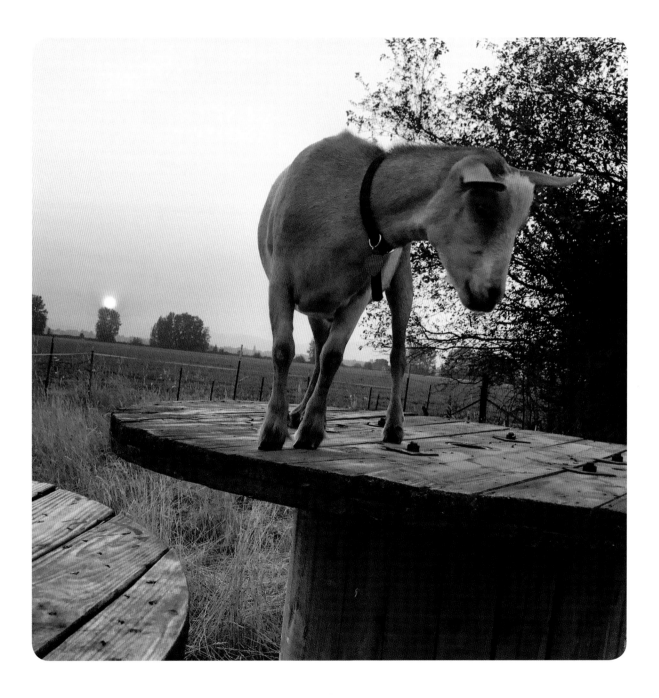

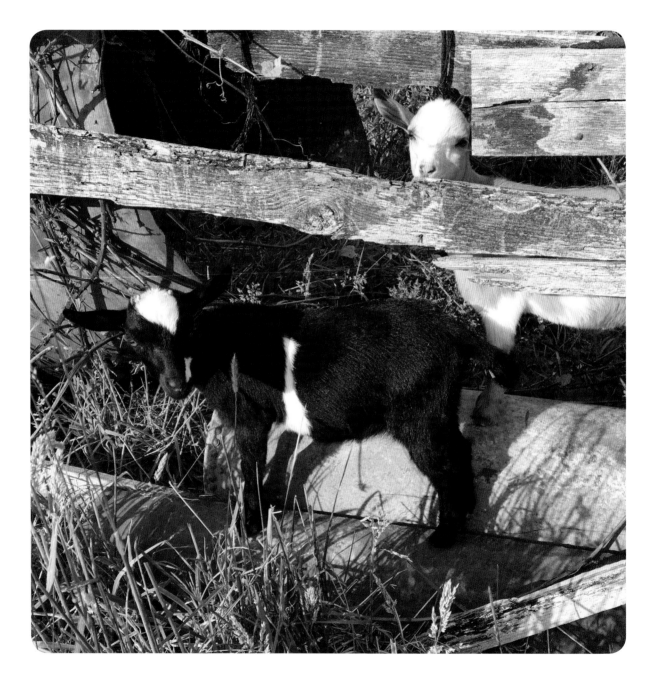

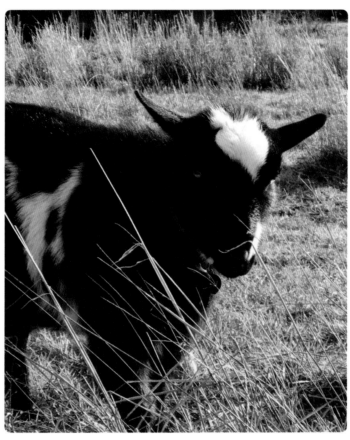

Quincy

I wonder which human belongs to those sneakers and if they'd notice if I took them . . .

Oh, hi! I'm Quincy. I would *never* steal anyone's shoes, but I *would* walk around a yoga class to make sure you were breathing deeply during Savasana. I may also jump on your back!

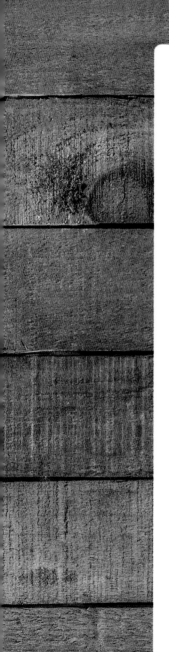

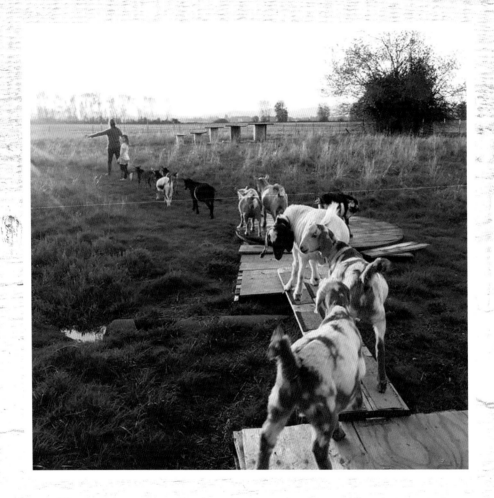

Them: This is so easy! Just follow our lead!

Us: That's what you said about spin class.

your
GOAT YOGA
practice

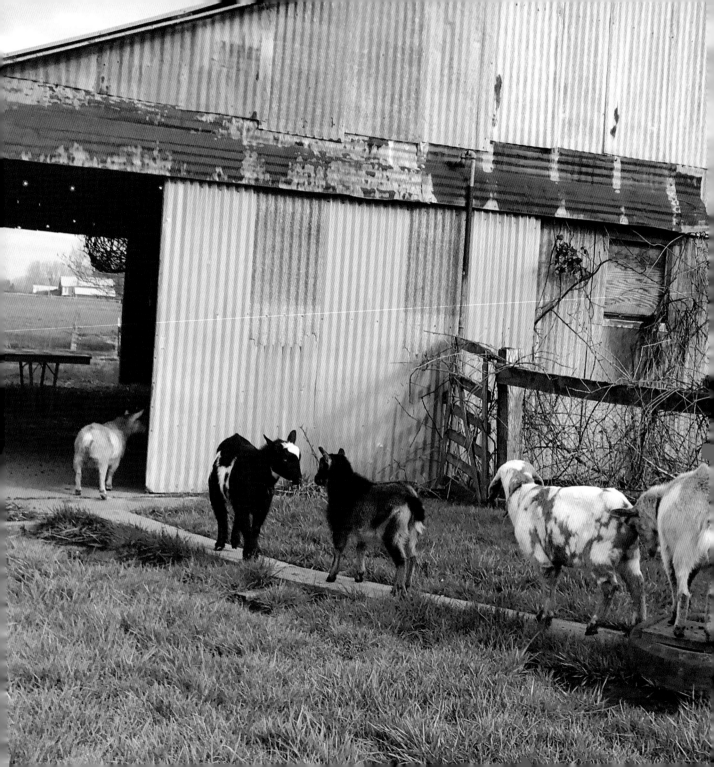

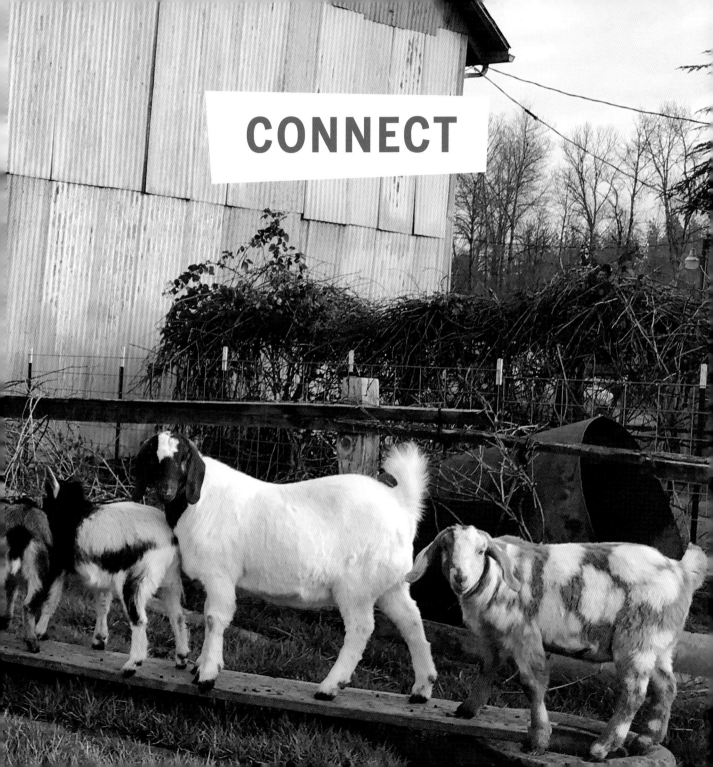

CONNECT

Mountain Pose

TADASANA

Stand at the top of your mat with your legs slightly spread and your feet planted firmly to the ground.

Acknowledge yourself.

Now bring your hands to heart center.

Close your eyes and take a few deep breaths in and out through your nose.

What do you notice?

Pay attention to how your body feels. Where is your breath?

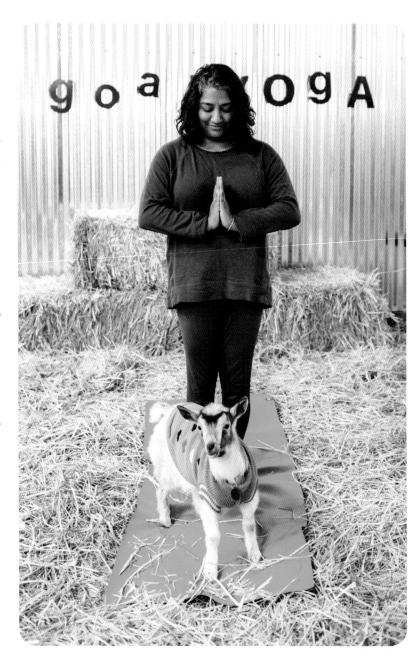

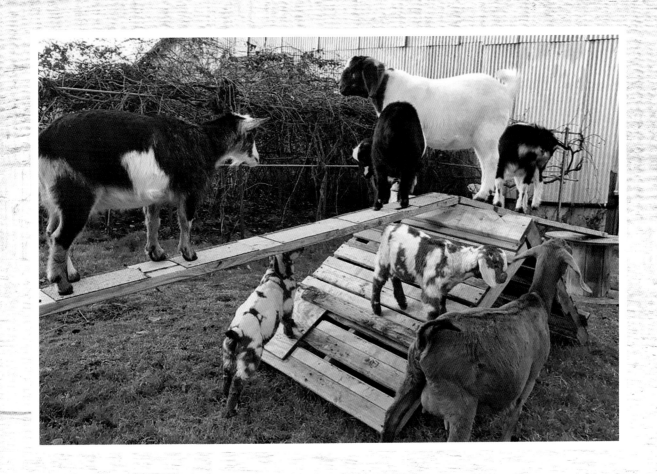

Are we doing it? Are we doing a yoga?

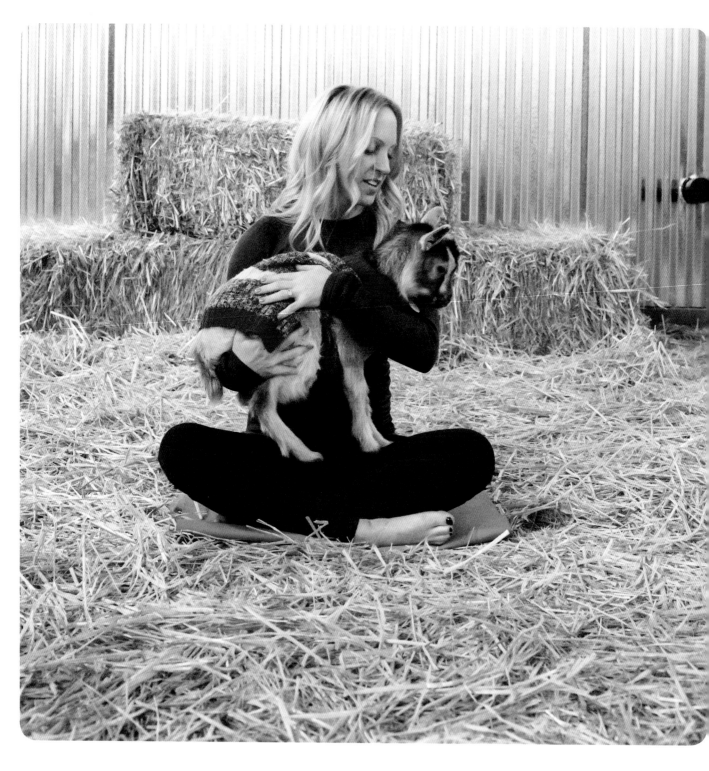

Seated Position

SUKHASANA

Fold a thick blanket or two into a firm support about 6 inches high, and place it under your bottom. Stretch your legs out in front of your torso on the floor.

Cross your shins, widen your knees, and slip each foot beneath your opposite knee as you bend your knees and fold your legs in toward your torso.

Relax your feet so their outer edges rest comfortably on the floor and your inner arches settle just below your opposite shin. You'll know you have the basic leg fold of *Sukhasana* when you look down and see a triangle, its three sides formed by your two thighs and your crossed shins. Don't confuse this position with the cross-legged position in which your ankles are tucked in close to your sitting bones. In *Sukhasana*, there should be a comfortable gap between your feet and pelvis.

You should sit with your pelvis in a relatively neutral position. To find neutral, press your hands against the floor and lift your sitting bones slightly off the support. As you hang there for a few breaths, make your thigh bones heavy, then slowly lower your sit bones lightly back to the support. Try to balance your pubic bone and tailbone so they're equidistant from the floor.

Either stack your hands in your lap, palms up, or lay your hands on your knees, palms down. Lengthen your tailbone toward the floor, firm your shoulder blades against your back to your upper torso, but be mindful not to overarch your lower back or poke your lower front ribs forward.

Take 8 breaths here to find your mindful breath and begin your practice.

NOTE If you practice this pose regularly, be sure to alternate the cross of your legs. A good rule of thumb: On even-numbered days, cross your right shin in front of your left, and on odd-numbered days, do the opposite. Alternately, you can divide the practice time in half, and spend the first half with your right leg forward and the second half with your left leg forward.

connect

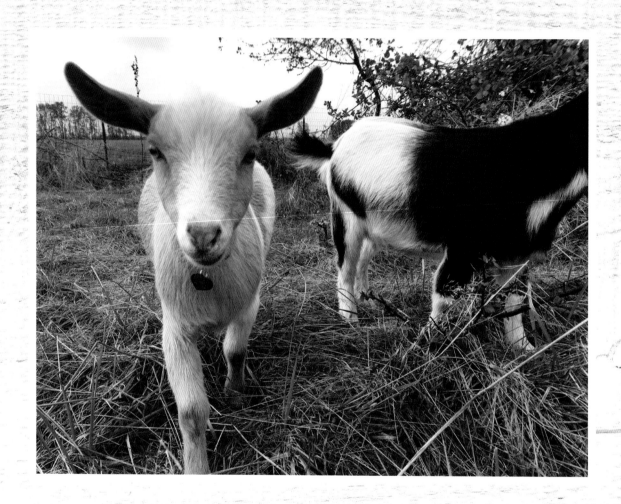

We already know how to breathe,
but we'd be happy to help you learn.

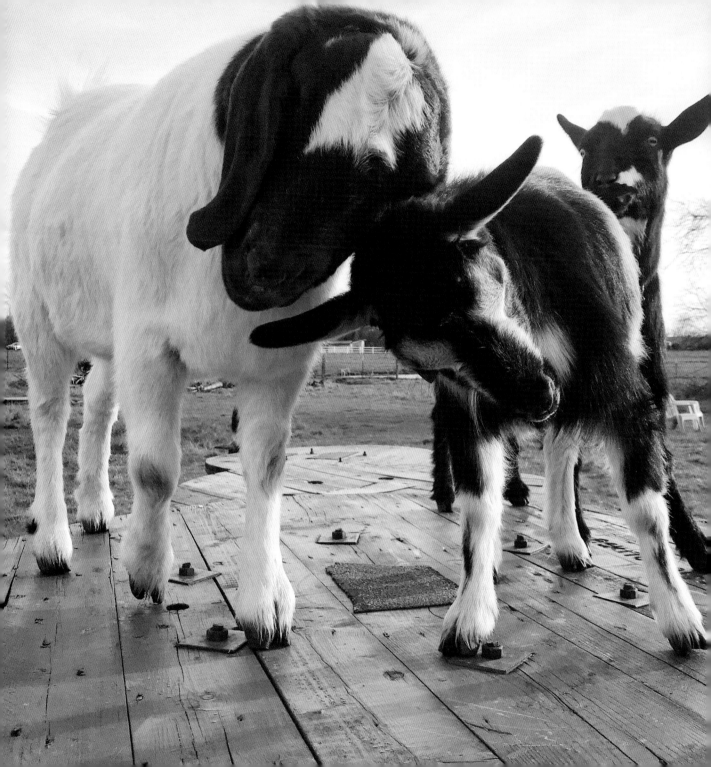

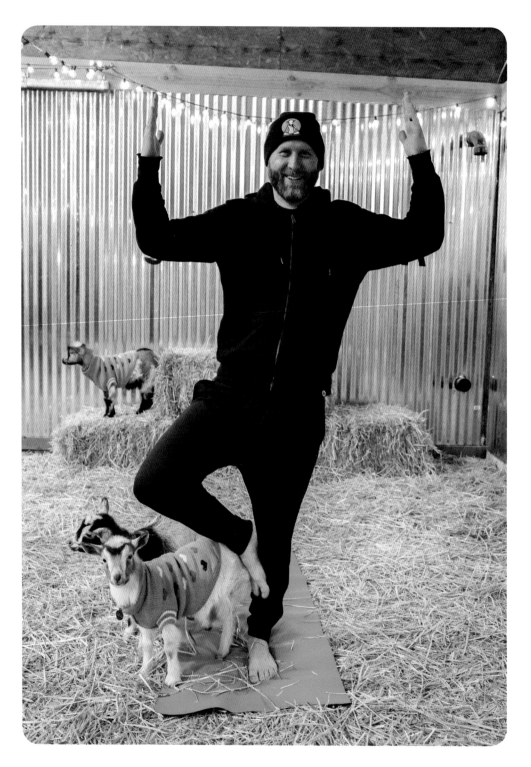

Tree Pose

VRKSASANA

Start in Mountain Pose. Transfer your weight onto your left leg, then bend your right knee, turn your right knee outward, and place the bottom of your right foot on the inside of your left ankle or calf.

Look down at the floor and stare at one point. Slowly slide your right foot up your left leg, only as high up as you can maintain your balance (just don't rest your foot on the inside of your left knee). When you are balanced here, slowly bring your palms together in a prayer position in front of your heart. Keep your left leg strong, pressing your foot into the floor and feeling your strength. Keep your right knee bent 90 degrees and pressing back. Move your shoulders down and back, and keep your chest pressing forward.

If you feel sturdy and it's accessible to you, try inhaling your arms over your head with your arms parallel in an "H" position, palms together with your thumbs crossed or fingers interlaced with your index finger pointed up. Feel your energy emanating skyward through your fingertips, but keep your shoulders down and back.

Breathe and hold for 4 to 8 breaths. To release, slowly exhale your arms down and come back into Mountain. Repeat on your other side.

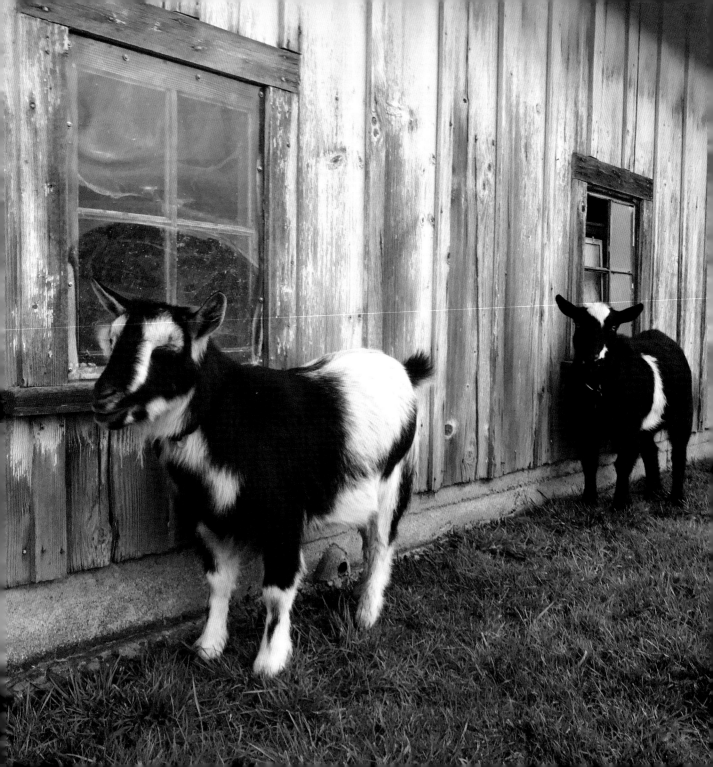

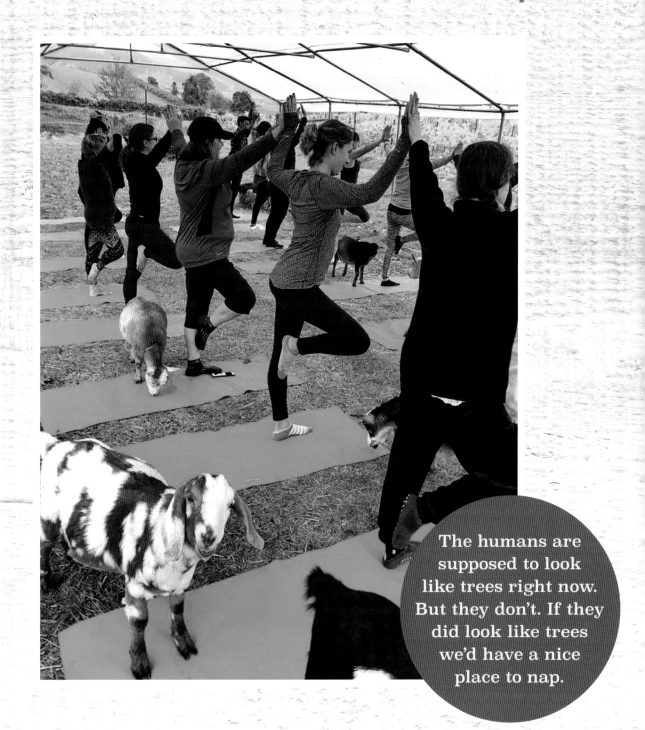

The humans are supposed to look like trees right now. But they don't. If they did look like trees we'd have a nice place to nap.

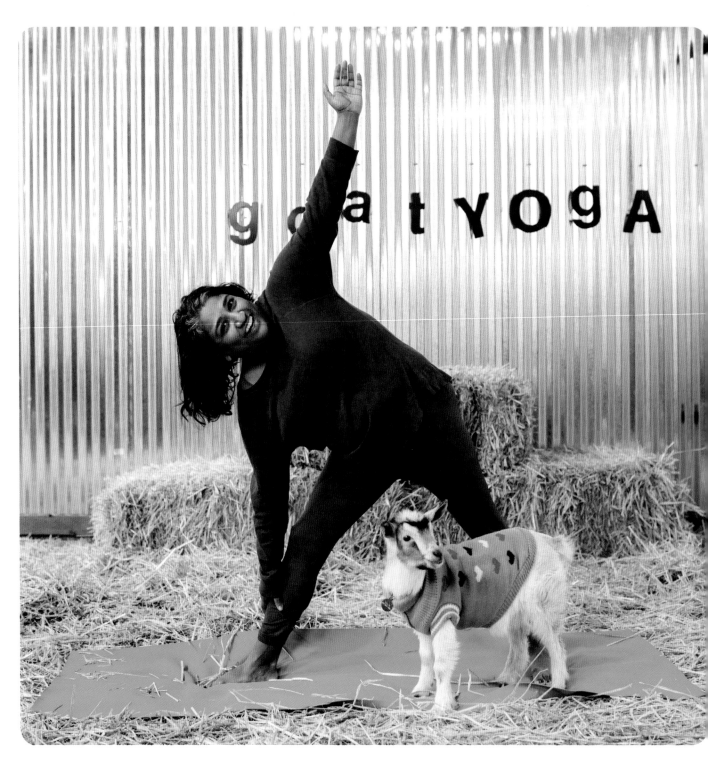

Extended Triangle

UTTHITA TRIKONASANA

Begin standing at the top of your mat in Mountain Pose (*Tadasana*). On an exhalation, step your left foot back about 3 to 4 feet (depending on the length of your legs and the level of openness in your hips and groins), placing it parallel to the back edge of your mat.

Angle your left foot in slightly (approximately 15 to 20 degrees), and line up the heel of your right foot with the heel of your left foot. With straight legs, firm your thighs without locking into your knees, and root the mound of your right big toe into your mat to activate and lift the arch of your front foot.

With an inhalation, extend your arms to shoulder height alongside your body, parallel to the floor with your palms facing down. Reach out actively through the fingertips of both hands and soften the tops of your shoulders.

Extend your right hand forward, and when you reach as far forward as you can while keeping your hips stationary, hinge at your right hip to bring your right hand down, keeping your front body and pelvis facing toward the left edge of your mat. If you have a block, place your right hand on a block just outside the pinky toe edge of your right foot—if a block isn't available, place your right hand lightly on your right shin for support.

Reach your left arm straight up toward the ceiling, firming your shoulder blades onto your back and broadening across your entire wingspan. Lengthen evenly through both sides of your torso, and press into the support under your right hand to grow taller through your left fingertips and broaden across your collarbone.

Root down evenly through the four corners of both feet, paying particular attention to the outer edge of your back foot, which has a tendency to collapse inward. Keep your head in a neutral position or send your gaze up toward your left hand if it feels comfortable for your neck.

Remain in the pose for 5 full breaths. On an inhalation, send your gaze down and press firmly into the soles of both feet to bring yourself back upright to stand, and step forward to the top of your mat. Reverse your feet and repeat.

connect

45

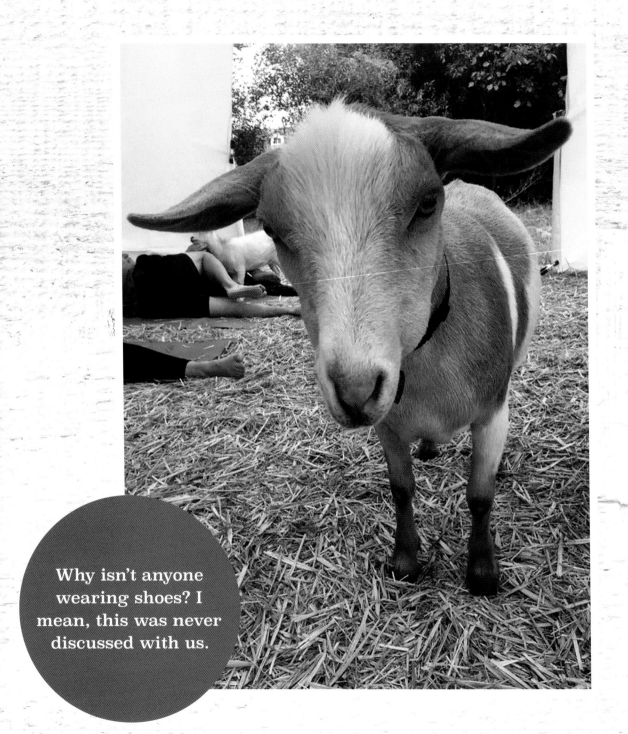

Why isn't anyone wearing shoes? I mean, this was never discussed with us.

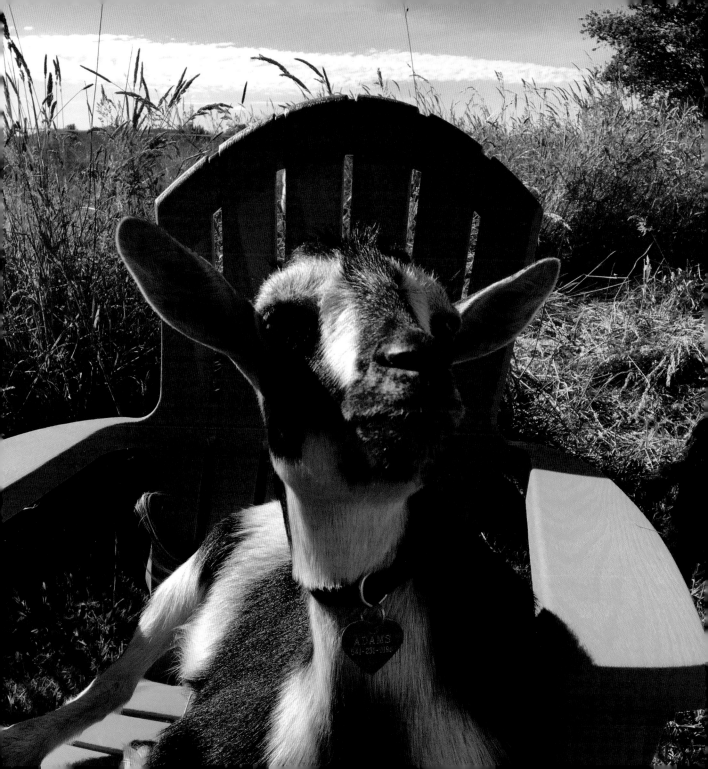

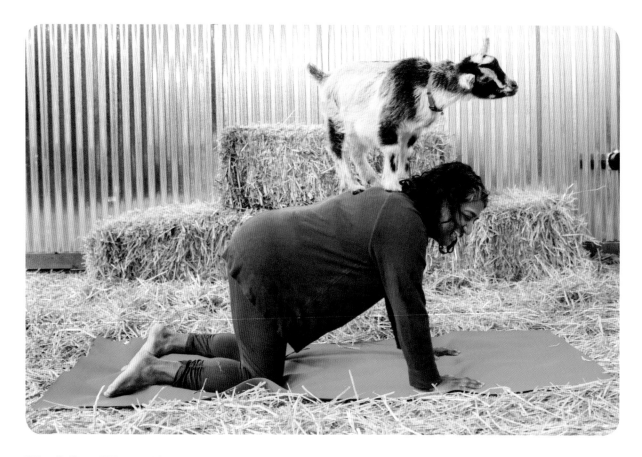

Table Top Pose

BHARMANASANA

Come to the floor on your hands and knees. Bring your knees hip-width apart with your feet directly behind your knees. Bring your palms directly under your shoulders with your fingers facing forward.

Look down between your palms and allow your back to be flat.

Press into your palms to drop your shoulders slightly away from your ears. Press your tailbone toward the back wall and the crown of your head toward the front wall to lengthen your spine.

Breathe deeply and hold for 1 to 3 breaths.

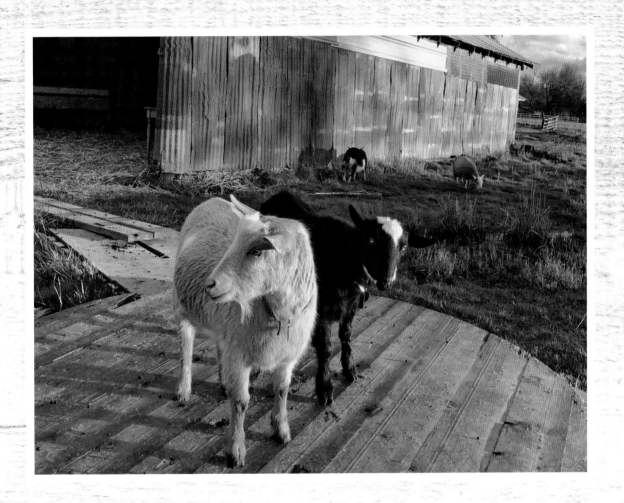

When I said I wanted table service,
this is not what I meant.

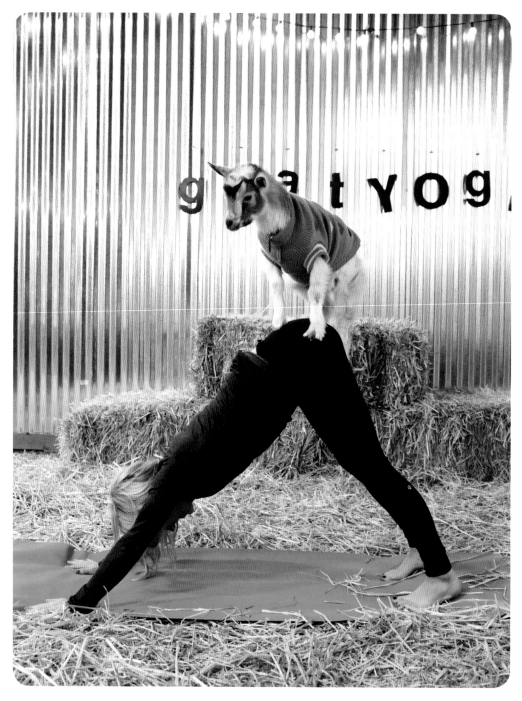

I have never seen any dogs do this.

Downward-Facing Dog Pose

ADHO MUKHA SVANASANA

From Table Top, exhale as you tuck your toes and lift your knees off the floor. Reach your pelvis up toward the ceiling, then gently begin to straighten your legs, but do not lock your knees. Bring your body into the shape of an upside-down letter "V." Imagine your hips and thighs being pulled backward from the top of your thighs, and press the floor away from you as you lift through your pelvis. As you lengthen your spine, lift your sit bones up toward the ceiling. Press down equally through your heels and the palms of your hands.

Firm the outer muscles of your arms, and press your index fingers into the floor. Lift from the inner muscles of your arms to the top of both shoulders.

Draw your chest toward your thighs as you continue to press the mat away from you, lengthening and decompressing your spine.

Engage your quadriceps. Rotate your thighs inward as you continue to lift your sit bones high. Sink your heels toward the floor.

Align your ears with your upper arms. Relax your head, but do not let it dangle. Gaze between your legs or toward your navel.

To release, exhale as you gently bend your knees and come back to your hands and knees.

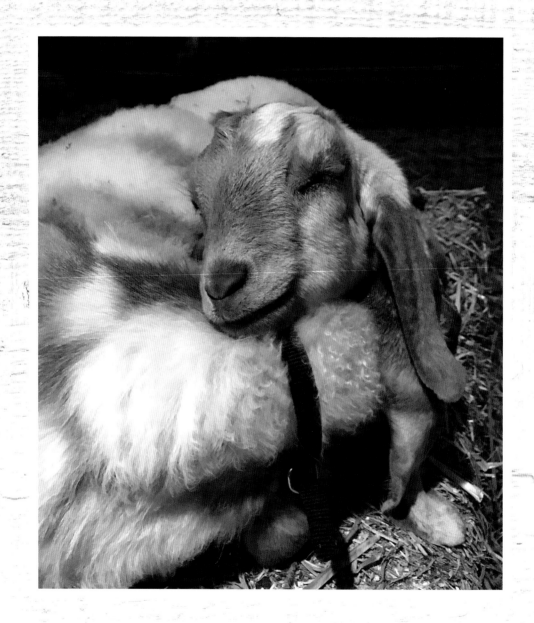

Yoga makes me sleepy.

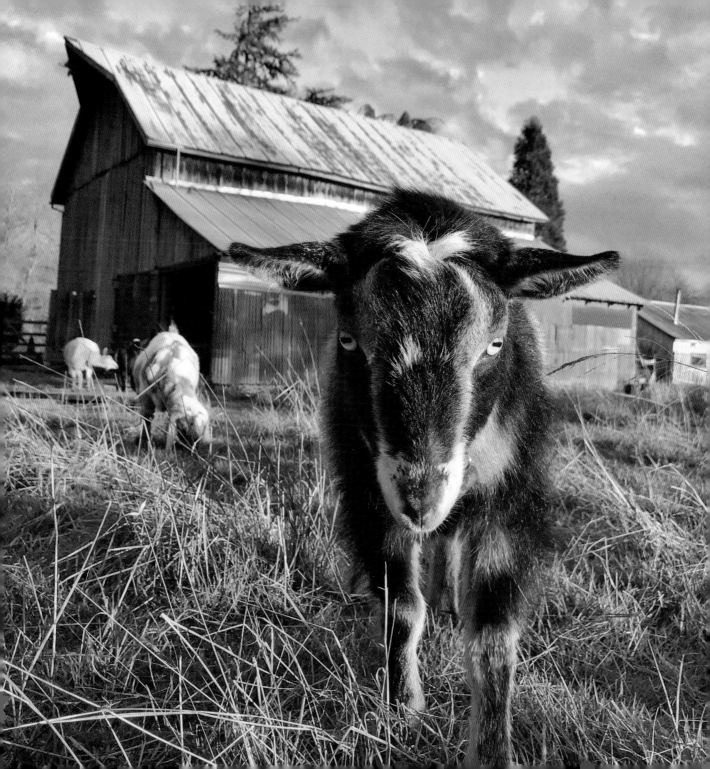

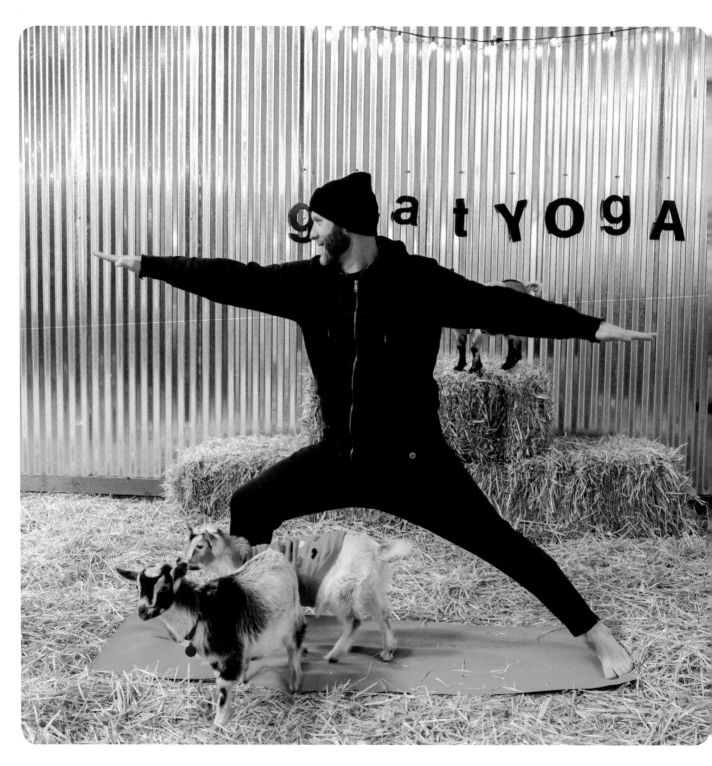

Warrior II Pose

VIRABHADRASANA II

Begin standing at the top of your mat in Mountain Pose. On an exhale, step your left foot back about 3 to 4 feet (depending on the length of your legs and the level of openness in your hips).

Place your left foot parallel to the short edge of your mat, and line up the heel of your right foot with the instep of your left foot. Press down firmly through the pinky toe edge of your back foot to avoid collapsing into the arch.

On an inhale, extend your arms with the right arm facing out in front of you and the left arm extending back, raising them parallel to the floor with your palms facing down. With soft eyes, send your gaze just over the middle finger of your right hand, and relax your shoulders down and away from your ears.

Bend deeply into your right knee, stacking it directly over your right ankle and bringing your right shin perpendicular to the floor. Ensure your knee isn't bowing out to the left or the right or extending past your toes.

Slightly scoop your tailbone under and open your pelvis to face the left side of your mat. Draw your low ribs into your body and keep your core gently engaged. Continue pressing through the pinky toe edge of your back foot, particularly through the outer edge of your heel.

Remain in the pose anywhere from 5 to 10 breaths. On an inhale, straighten your front leg and exhale to lower your arms. Step to the front of your mat, and repeat on the other side whenever you feel ready.

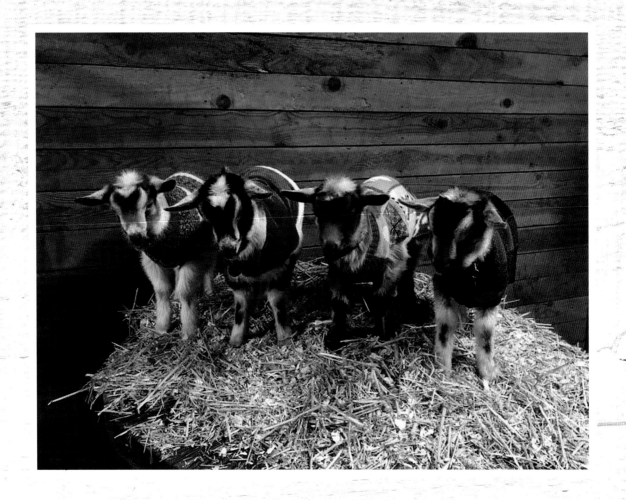

We even called each other to make sure no one
would wear the same sweater as anyone else.
Dangit.

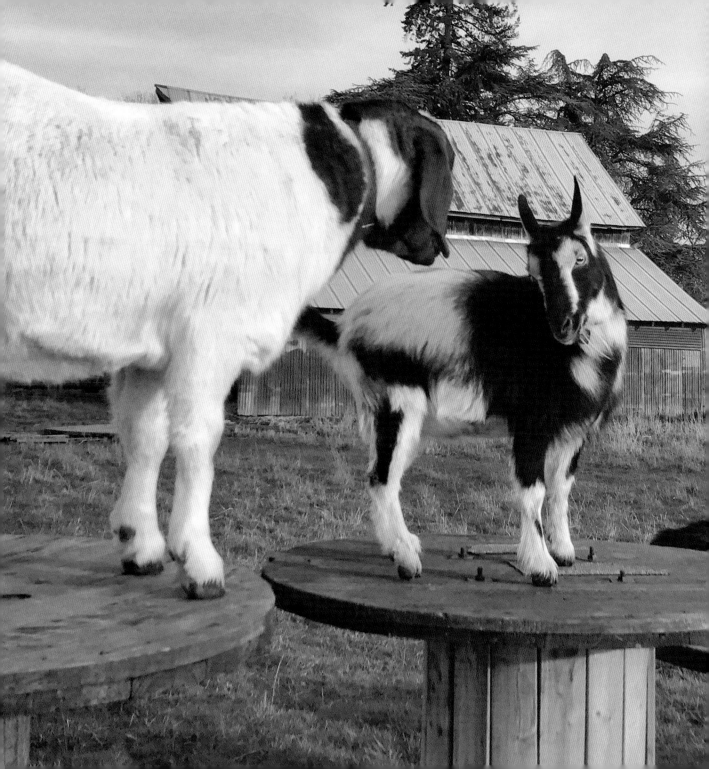

Cobra Pose

BHUJANGASANA

Lie on your stomach with your legs straight behind you and the tops of your feet on the floor. Hugging your elbows to your ribs, place your hands on the floor directly under your shoulders. Press the tops of your feet, thighs, and pubis firmly into the floor.

On an inhalation, begin to straighten your arms to lift your chest off the floor, going only to the height at which you can maintain a connection through your pubis to your legs. Press your tailbone toward your pubis, and lift your pubis toward your navel. Narrow your hip points.

Firm your shoulder blades against your back, puffing your side ribs forward. Lift through the top of your sternum, but avoid pushing your front ribs forward, which only hardens your lower back.

Distribute the backbend evenly throughout your entire spine.

Hold the pose anywhere from 5 to 10 breaths, breathing easily. Release back to the floor with an exhalation.

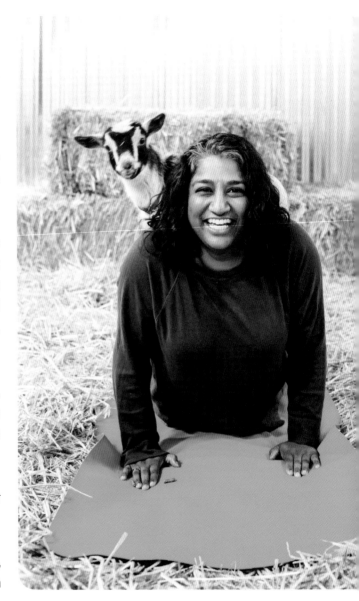

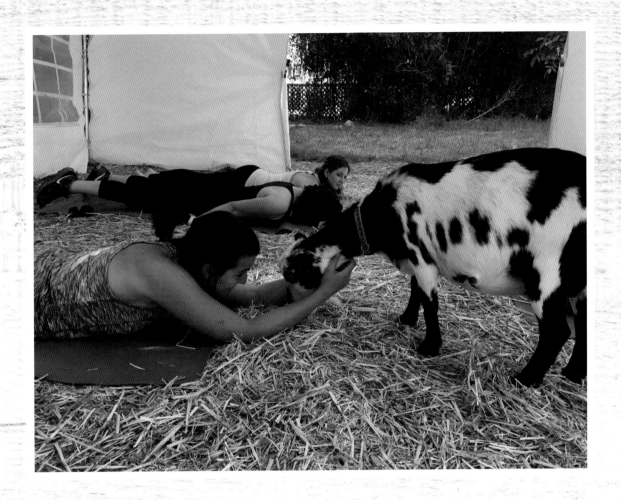

Hey! You look pretty nice for a cobra! What's that? Oh. "Cobra" is a yoga position. Got it.

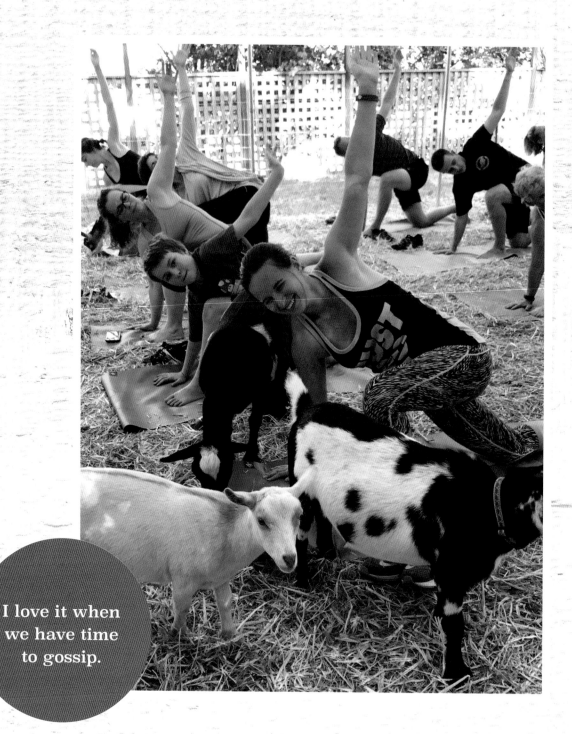

I love it when we have time to gossip.

High Lunge Pose

UTTHITA ASHWA SANCHALANASANA

On your hands and knees in Table Pose, step your right foot forward between your two hands, with your knee directly over your ankle. Tuck your back toes under and straighten your back leg (see pages 62 and 63).

Press your palms, fingers, or fists into the floor to lift the crown of your head up toward the ceiling. Roll your shoulders down and back, and press your chest forward. Look straight ahead with your chin parallel to the floor.

Extend your back leg by pressing your heel toward the floor and by pressing the back of your knee up toward the ceiling. Relax your hips and let them sink toward the floor.

Breathe and hold for 2 to 6 breaths.

Release by lowering your left knee and sliding your right knee back into Table Top. Alternatively, you can step your right foot back into Downward-Facing Dog.

Repeat on the other side.

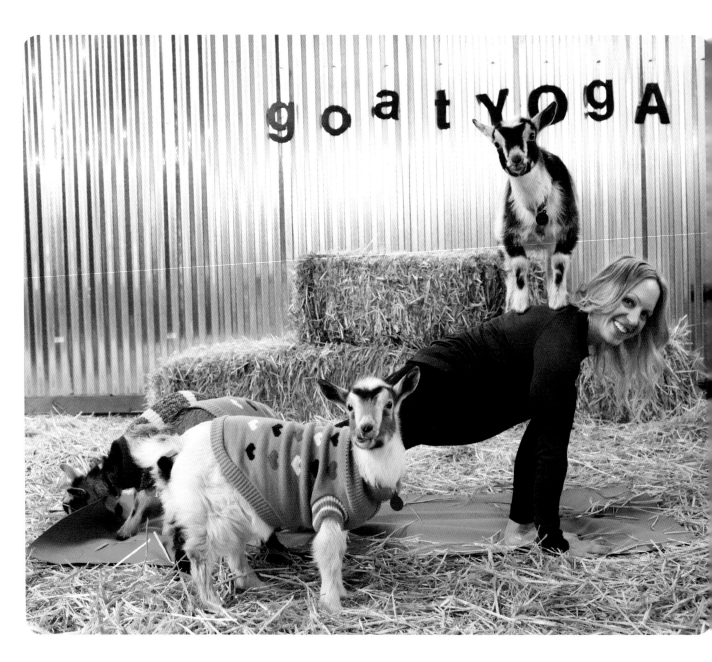

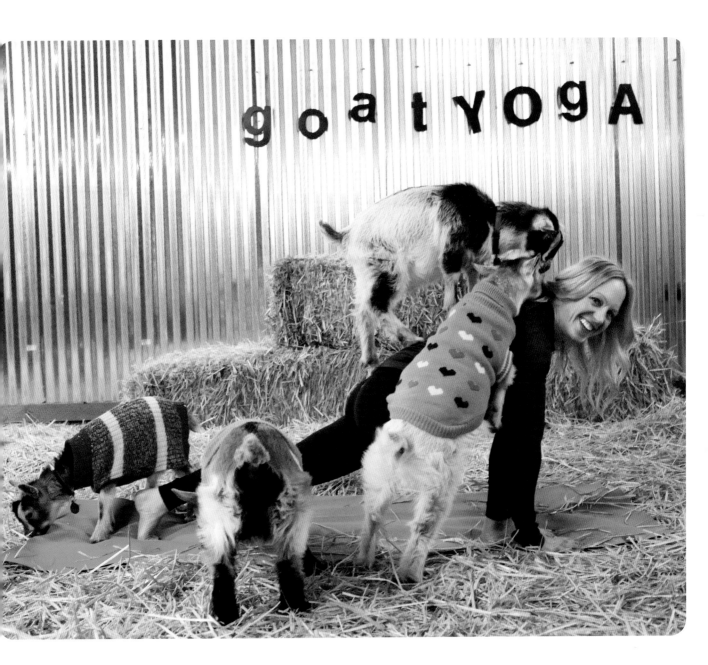

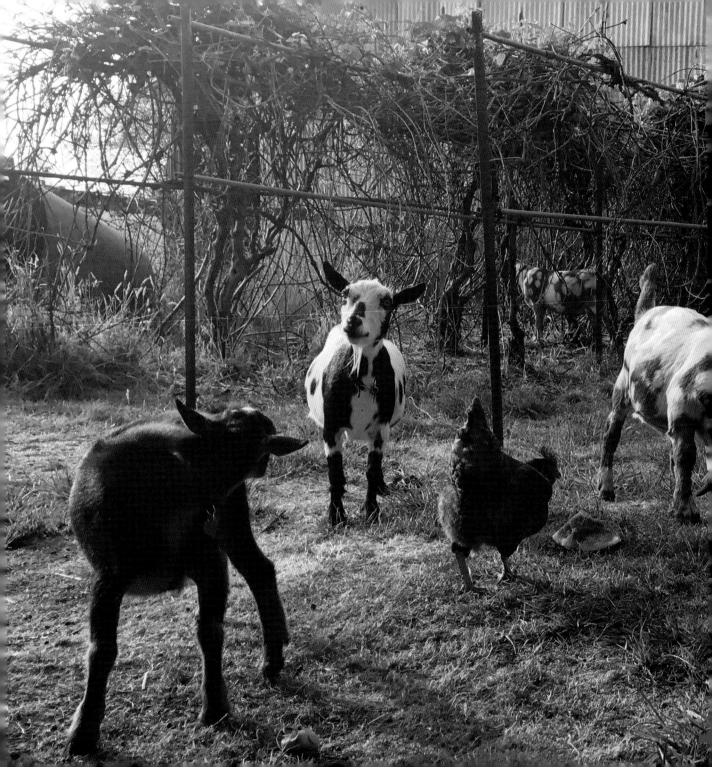

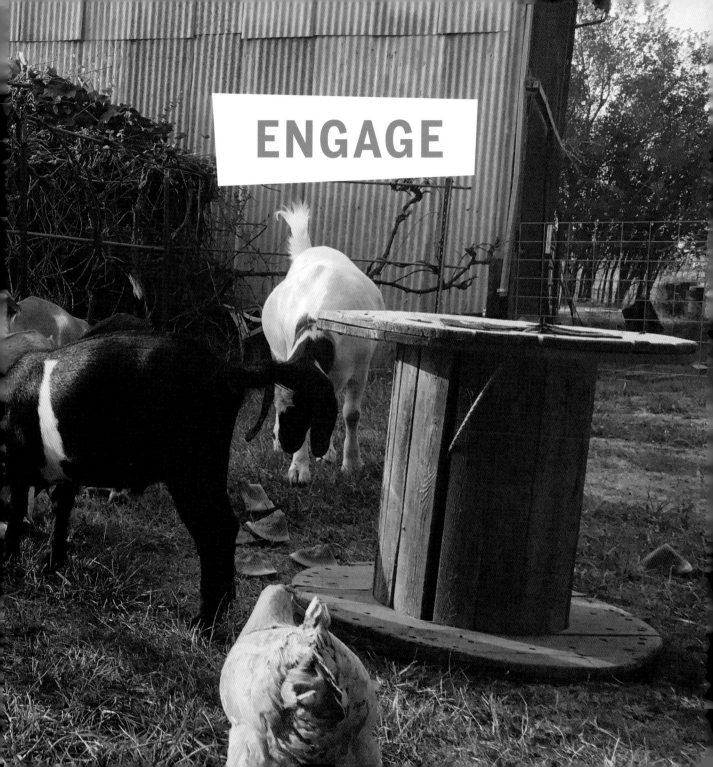

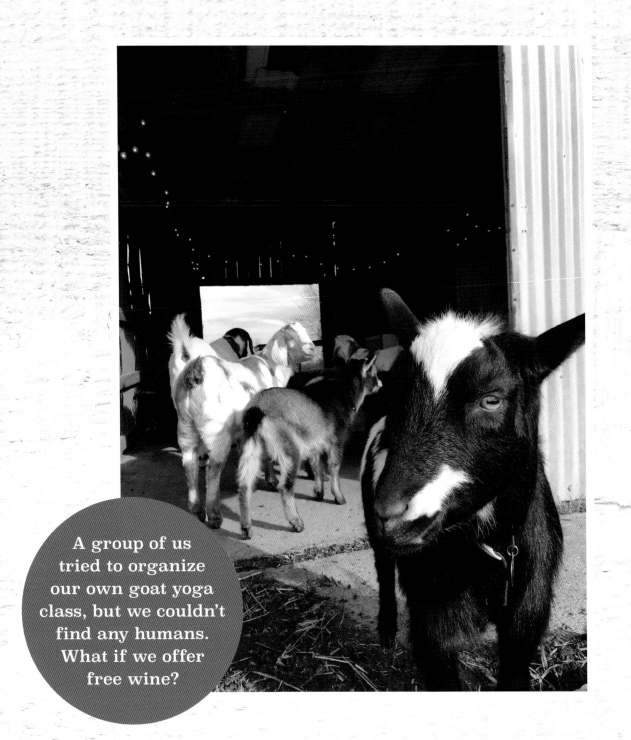

A group of us tried to organize our own goat yoga class, but we couldn't find any humans. What if we offer free wine?

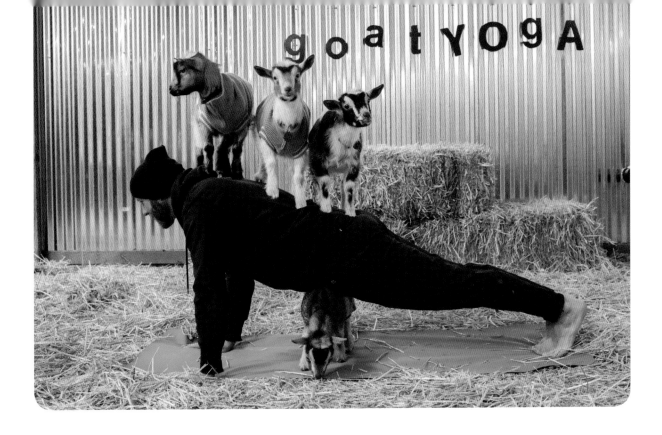

Plank Pose

KUMBHAKASANA

From Table Top, step or jump both feet back into a push-up position.

Spread your fingers wide apart with your middle finger pointing forward. Press into your palms with your arms straight. Tuck your tailbone under so your legs, hips, and torso are one straight line. Press the crown of your head forward, and with your toes tucked, press your heels back.

Breathe and hold for 1 to 4 breaths.

To release, either bend your knees to the floor into Child Pose, or bend your elbows and lower yourself into low plank.

engage

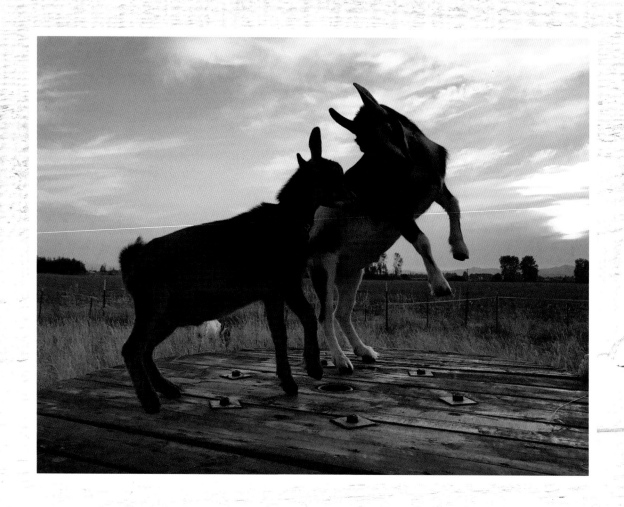

I've invented a new yoga position.
I can't wait to demonstrate it in class.
The humans will love it.

Three-Legged Downward-Facing Dog Pose

TRI PADA ADHO MUKHA SVANASANA

Begin in Table Top Pose. Look down at your hands. Ensure that the creases of your wrists are parallel to the short edge of the mat, that your fingers are spread wide, and that your weight is distributed evenly through your palms and knuckles, particularly those of your pointer and middle finger.

On an exhale, tuck your toes under and begin to slowly extend your legs, lifting your hips high toward the ceiling. Keep your knees bent for as long as you need to in order to maintain the length along your spine.

Continue lifting your hips high and back, and press the tops of your thighs toward the back of the room. Keep your ears in line with your arms, and firm up through your upper outer arm.

On an inhale, extend your right leg up high and back, lifting it toward the ceiling (see page 70). Avoid the tendency to tilt your pelvis and open up through your hips in an effort to lift your leg as high as possible; rather, keep your hips level and your right foot flexed (with your heel reaching back and your toes pointing toward the ground).

You can remain here with your hips level if this feels like enough, or, to move even deeper, begin to bend your right knee so that your foot drops over to the left. Point your bent knee toward the ceiling, and begin to open up and stack your hips directly on top of one another (see page 71).

Your weight will want to shift into your left side here. Keep your weight evenly distributed across both palms, and drop your right shoulder so that your upper body remains squared.

Stay in the pose for 5 to 10 breaths, then slowly square off your hips and lower your extended leg on an exhale. Gently walk out your legs in Downward-Facing Dog, then repeat on your other side.

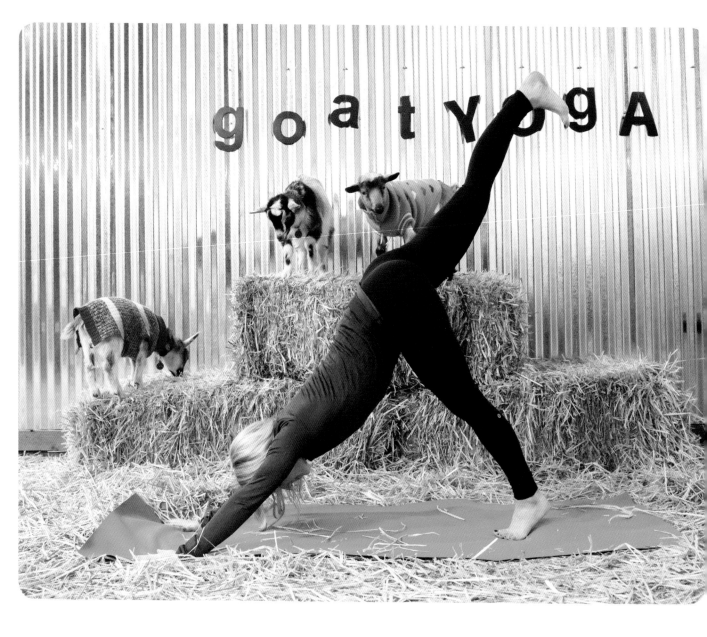

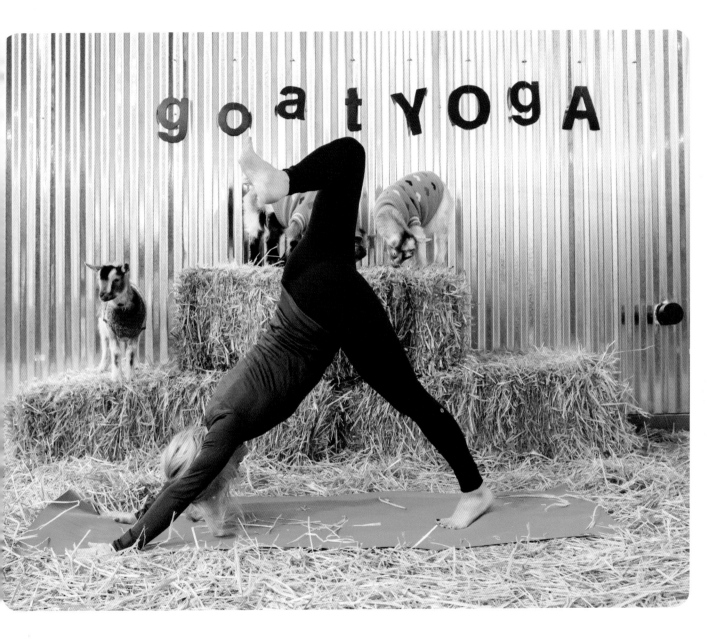

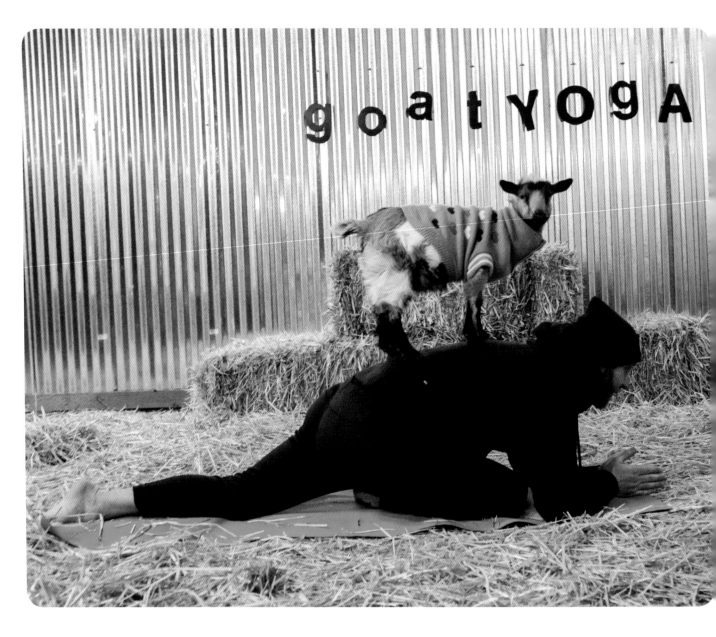

Pigeon Pose

EKA PADA RAJAKAPOTASANA

Begin in Downward-Facing Dog. On an exhale, bend your right knee into your chest, and gently lower your bent right knee to meet the outside of your right wrist.

Move your right shin parallel to the short edge of your mat (your right foot will move toward your left wrist) until you find an angle that feels appropriate for your body.

Lower your left leg onto the mat and extend it straight behind you. Keep the top of your left foot relaxed on the mat.

Place your fingertips on the ground beside your hips, and square your hips forward to the front of the room. Note the tendency for your right hip to drop here; instead, focus on maintaining an even distribution of weight across both hips.

Inhale here, lengthening your spine and reaching the crown of your head toward the ceiling.

Walk your fingertips in front of your right shin, coming down onto your palms, forearms, or folding forward and resting your forehead on the tops of your hands.

Stay in the pose anywhere from 10 to 20 breaths depending on your comfort level. The longer the pose is held, the more your muscles around your joints will relax and begin to stretch and lengthen.

To come out of the pose, plant your palms on the mat in front of you, and slowly make your way back to Downward-Facing Dog (it doesn't have to look pretty!). Bend your knees one at a time, gently walking out your legs. Whenever you feel ready, repeat the pose on your other side.

engage

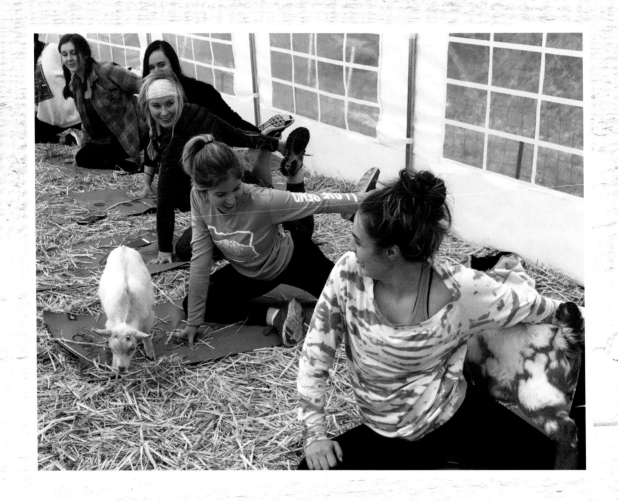

Last we heard, pigeons were birds. These are not birds. They are humans pretending to be birds. We are goats pretending to believe the humans are pigeons.

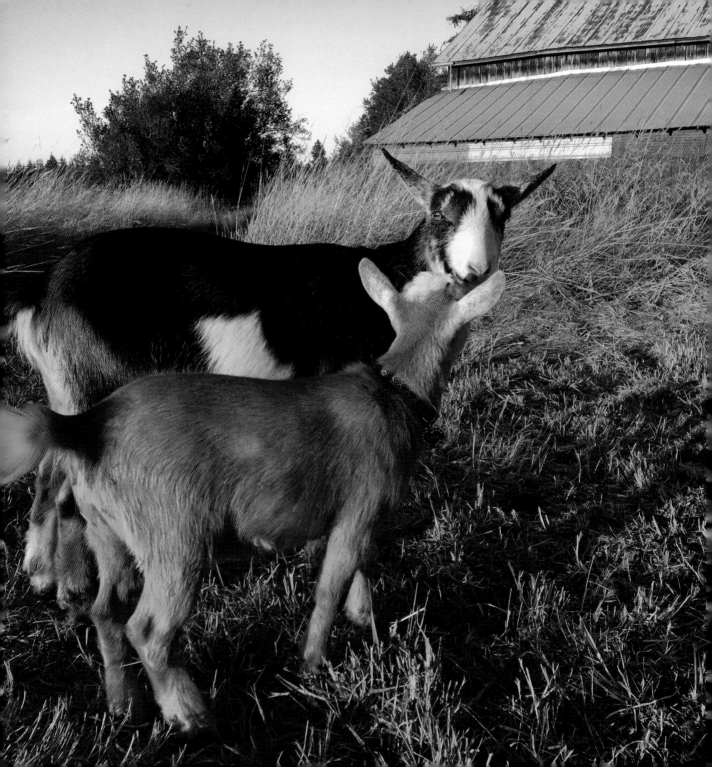

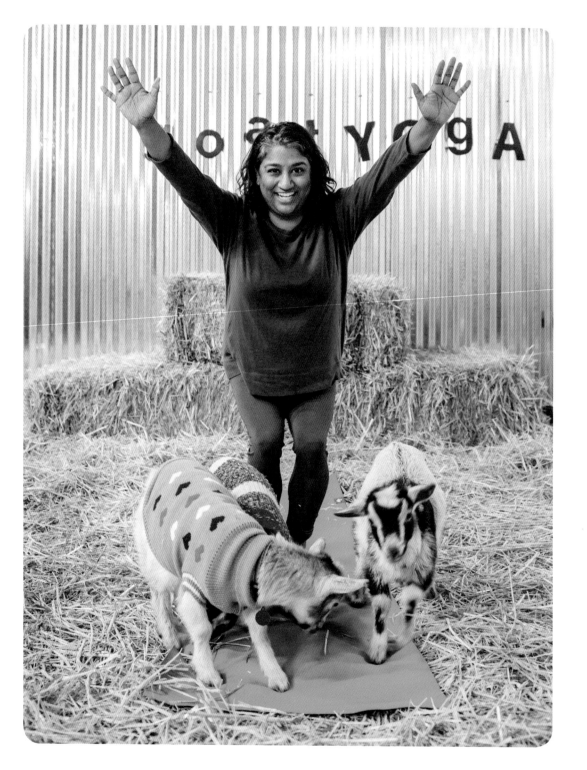

Chair Pose

UTKATASANA

Stand with your feet together and your big toes touching. Beginners can stand with their feet hip-distance apart.

Inhale and raise your arms above your head, perpendicular to the floor.

Exhale as you bend your knees, bringing your thighs as parallel to the floor as they can get. Your knees will project slightly over your feet, and your torso will form an approximate right angle over your thighs.

Draw your shoulder blades into your upper back ribs as you reach your elbows back toward your ears. Do not puff your rib cage forward. Draw your tailbone down to the floor, keeping your lower back long.

Bring your hips down even lower, and lift through your heart. There will be a slight bend in your upper back.

Shift your weight into your heels. Transfer enough weight—approximately 80 percent—to your heels so that you could lift your toes off the mat if you wanted to.

Keep your breath smooth, even, and deep. If your breath becomes shallow or strained, back off a bit in the pose until breathing becomes easier.

Spread your shoulder blades apart. Spin your pinky fingers toward each other so your palms face each other, rotating your arms outward through your thumbs.

Gaze directly forward. For a deeper pose, tilt your head slightly and gaze at a point between your hands.

Hold for up to 5 breaths Then, inhale as you straighten your legs, lifting through your arms. Exhale and release.

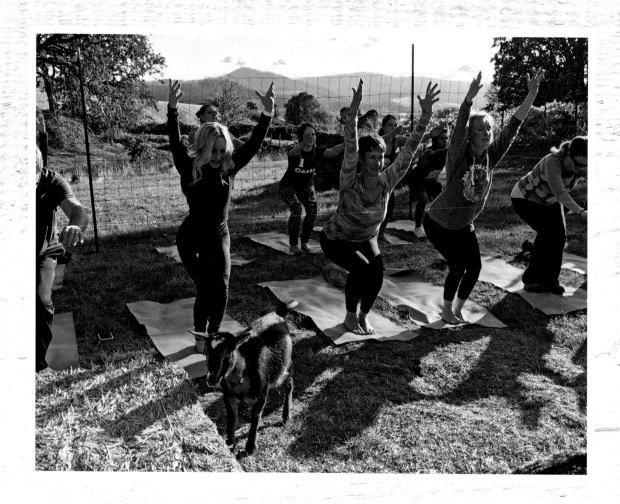

Where are the chairs?

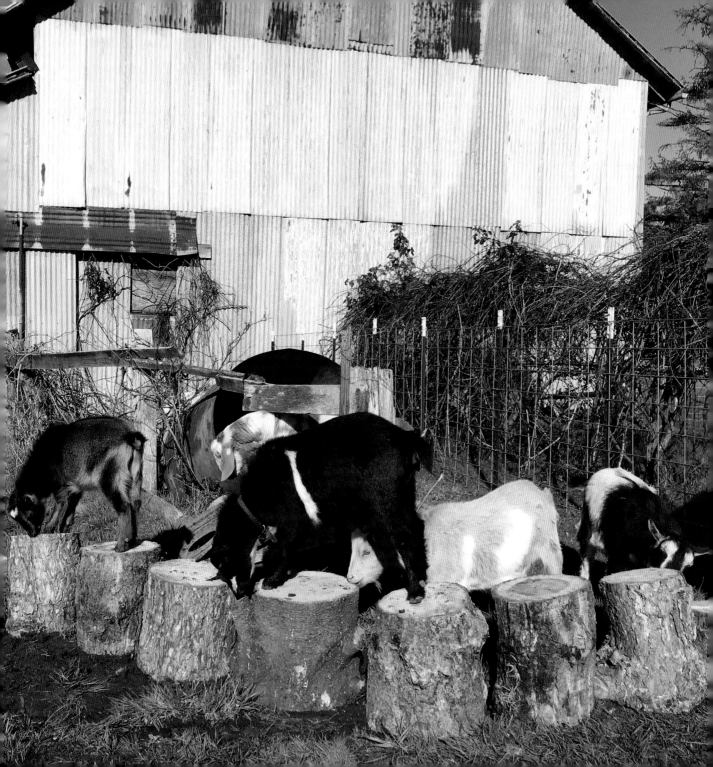

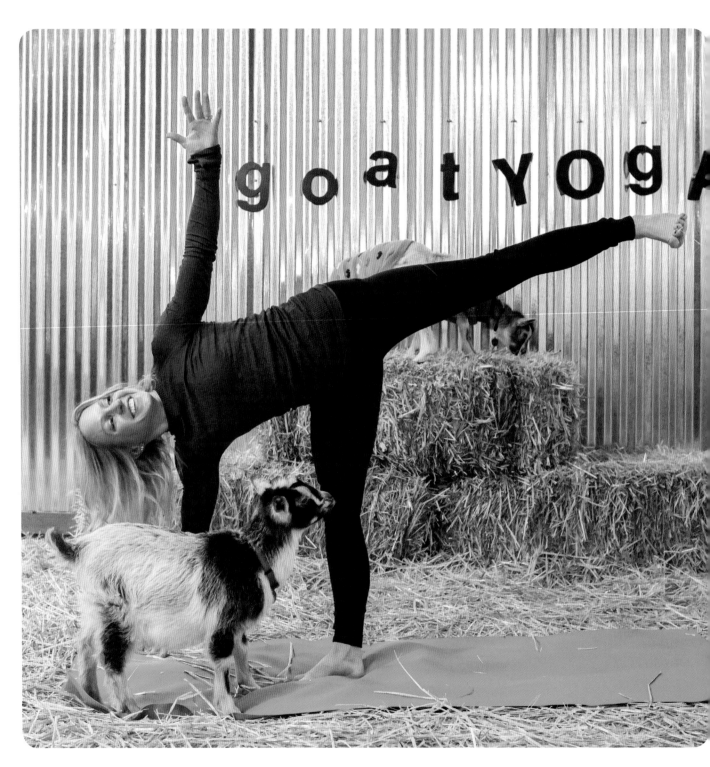

Half Moon Pose

ARDHA CHANDRASANA

Begin by standing at the top of your mat. Turn to the left and step your feet wide apart. Extend your arms out to your sides at shoulder height. Your feet should be as far apart as your wrists. Rotate your right (front) foot 90 degrees so your front foot's toes point to the top of the mat. Turn your left foot's toes slightly in. Align your front heel with the arch of your back foot.

Reach through your right hand in the same direction that your right foot is pointed. Shift your left hip back, and then fold sideways at the hip. Rest your right hand on your outer right shin or ankle. If you are more flexible, place your fingertips on the floor. You can also place your hand on a yoga block.

Align your shoulders so your left shoulder is directly above your right shoulder. Gently turn your head to gaze at your left thumb.

Bring your left hand to rest on your left hip. Turn your head to look at the floor. Then, bend your right knee and step your left foot 6 to 12 inches closer to your right foot. Place your right hand's fingertips on the floor in front of your right foot.

Press firmly into your right hand and foot. Straighten your right leg while simultaneously lifting your left leg. Work toward bringing your left leg parallel to the floor or even higher than your hips.

Reach actively through your left heel. Do not lock your right knee. Keep your right foot's toes and kneecap facing in the direction of your head.

Stack your top hip directly over your bottom hip, and open your torso to the left. Then extend your left arm and point your fingertips directly toward the sky. If you can balance comfortably there, turn your head and gaze at your left thumb.

Draw your shoulder blades firmly into your back. Lengthen your tailbone toward your left heel.

Hold for up to 5 breaths. To release, lower your left leg as you exhale. Return to Extended Triangle Pose. Inhale and press firmly through your left heel as you lift your torso. Lower your arms. Turn to the left, reversing the position of your feet, and repeat for the same length of time on the opposite side.

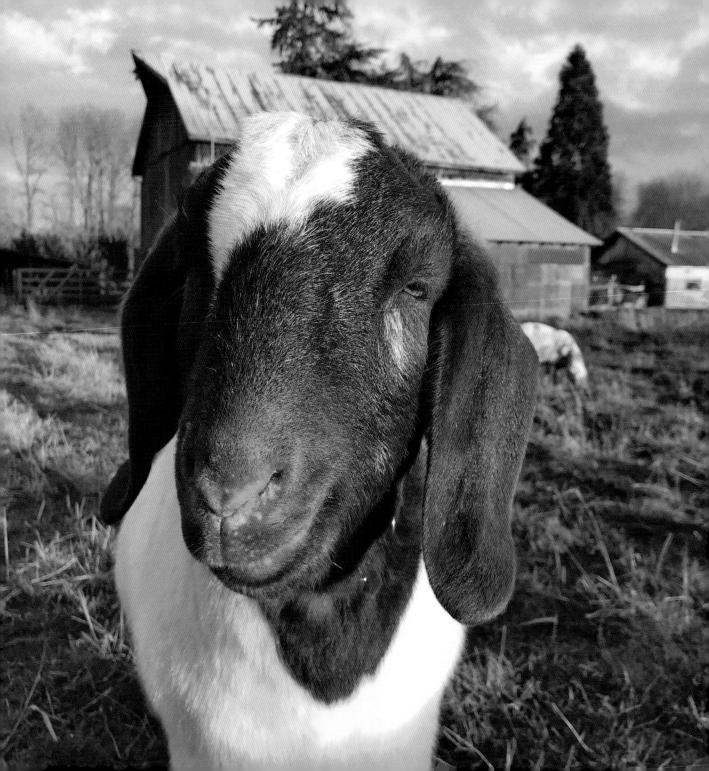

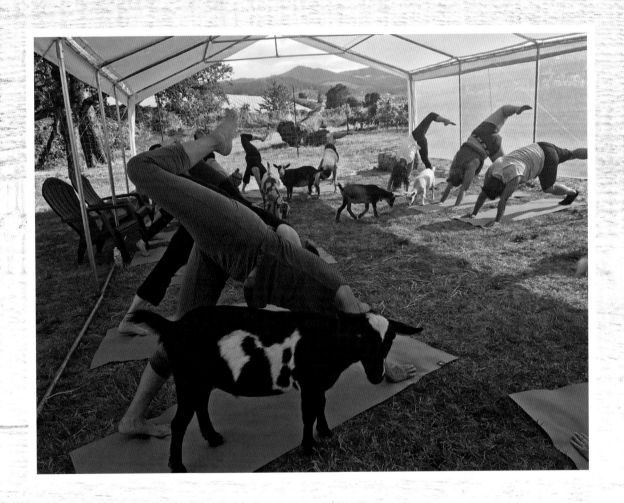

My legs don't bend that way.

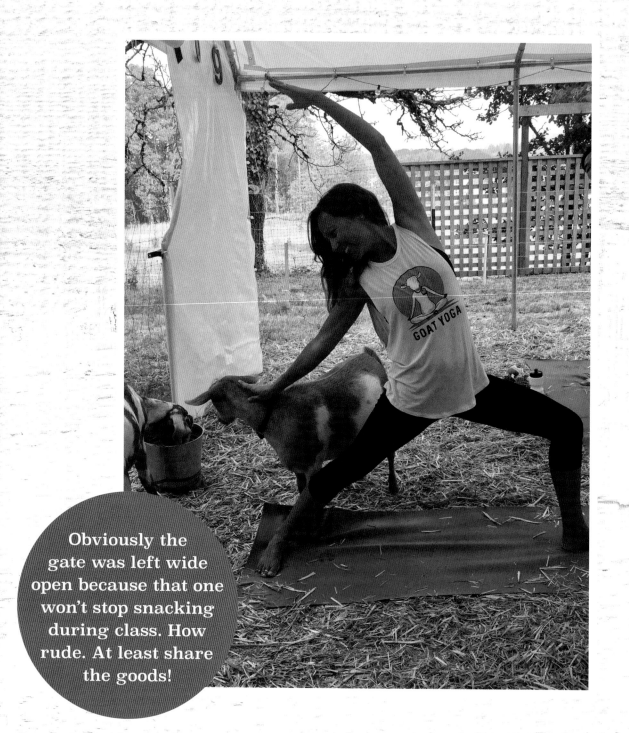

Obviously the gate was left wide open because that one won't stop snacking during class. How rude. At least share the goods!

Gate Pose

PARIGHASANA

Begin kneeling on the floor with your hips and buttocks lifted up off your legs. Place a folded blanket beneath your knees, shins, and feet if you need the extra padding to feel more comfortable. Your inner knees should be together, and your thighs should be perpendicular to the floor.

Extend your right leg out to the side. Keep your leg in line with your body (see page 86). Point your toes to the right with your kneecap pointing to the ceiling. Try to press the sole of your right foot all the way onto the floor while keeping your leg straight. Your pelvis will turn slightly to the right. Keep your upper torso turning against that pull to face forward.

On an inhale, extend your arms out to the sides to shoulder height with your palms facing down.

Rest your right hand along your right thigh, shin, or ankle. Turn your left palm upward, and then extend it toward the ceiling. Then reach your left arm overhead and to the right, so your bicep rests against your left ear. Turn your gaze toward the ceiling (see page 87).

Keep moving your left hip slightly forward and turning your torso away from the floor.

Hold for up to 10 breaths. To release, inhale as you lift through your left arm to draw your torso upright, keeping both arms extended. Lower your arms and move your right knee next to your left to regain balance. Repeat the pose for the same amount of time on the opposite side.

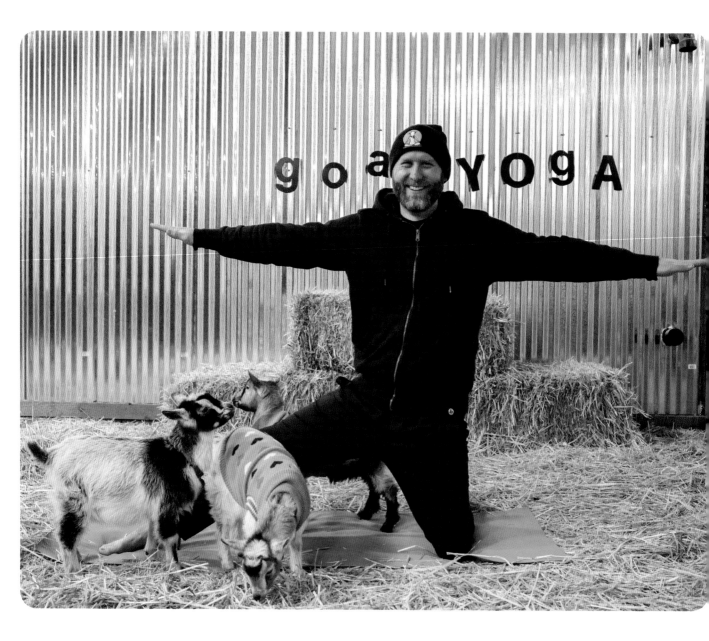

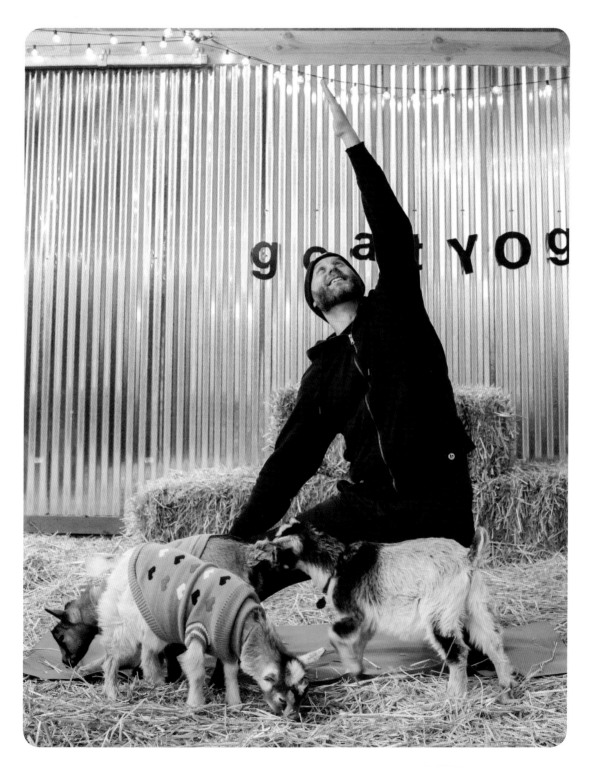

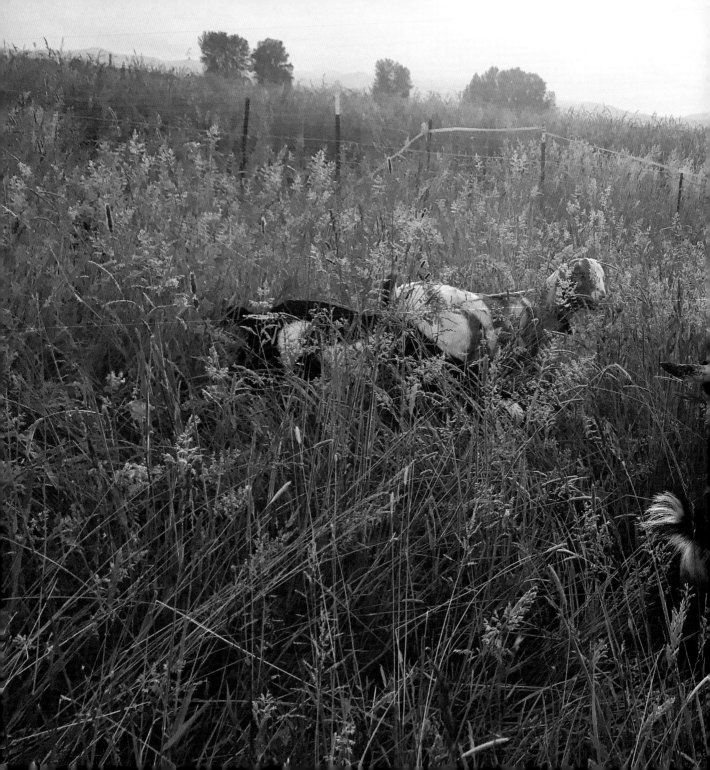

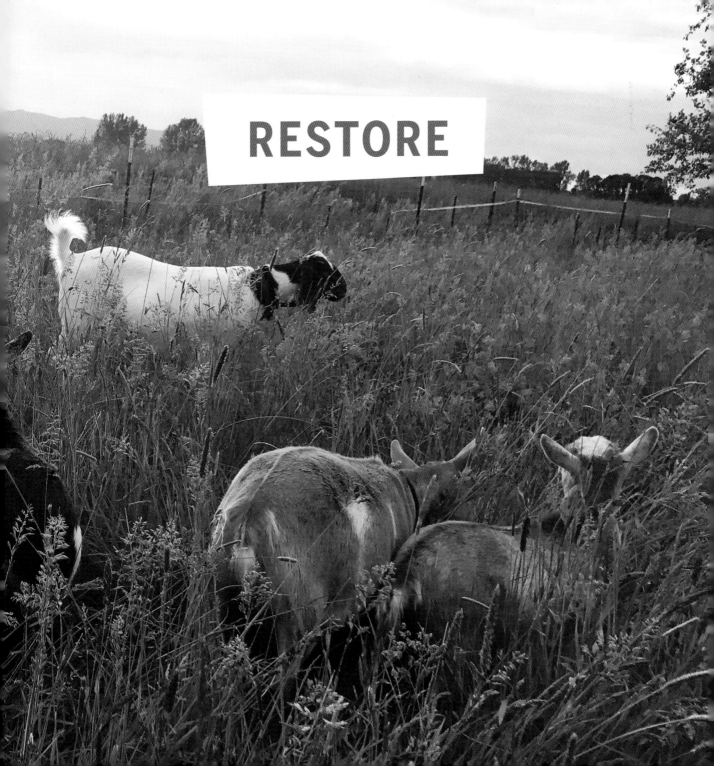

RESTORE

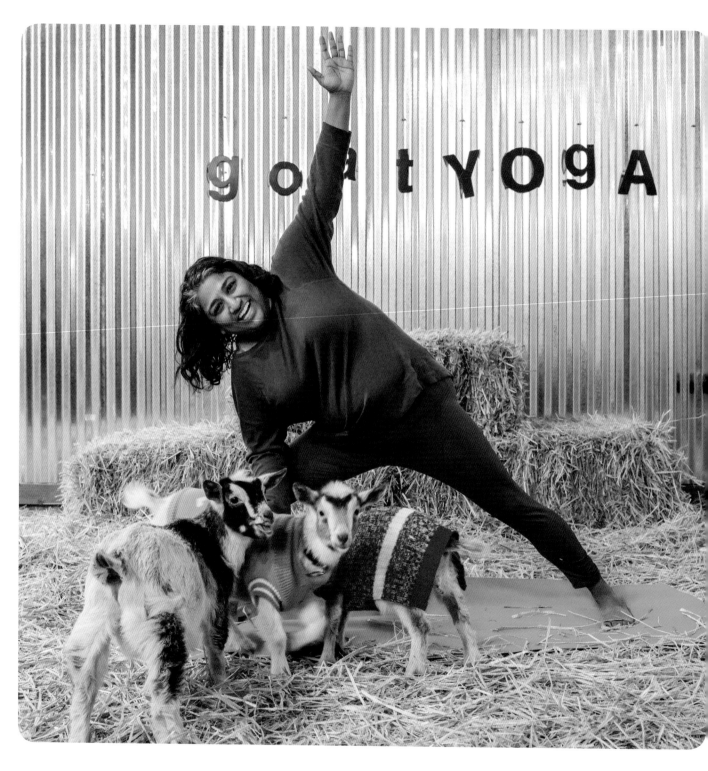

Extended Side Angle Pose

UTTHITA PARSVAKONASANA

Begin in Mountain Pose. Turn to the left, and extend your arms sideways to shoulder height, palms facing down. Step your feet as wide apart as your wrists. Align your heels.

Turn your right leg and foot outward 90 degrees so your toes point to the top of your mat. Bend your right knee until your right thigh is parallel to the floor (you may need to widen your stance). Keep your right knee directly over your heel. Slightly turn in your left toes. Align the heel of your right foot with the arch of your left foot. Keep your back leg straight. Inhale and draw your left hip slightly forward.

Keep your torso open to the left; do not turn your body in the direction of your right leg. Gaze out across the top of your right middle finger. Make sure your front knee does not drop inward. Keep your front thigh externally rotating with your knee drawn slightly toward the baby toe of your front foot. Press firmly through the outer edge of your back foot.

Exhaling, lower your right arm so your forearm rests on your right thigh.

Reach your left arm toward the ceiling, and then extend your arm over the top of your head. Your left bicep should be over your left ear, and your fingertips should be reaching in the same direction your front toes are pointing. Keep your chest, hips, and legs in one straight line, extended over your front leg.

Turn your head to look at the ceiling. Keep your throat soft and your breathing smooth. Relax your face.

To deepen the pose, lower your front hand to the floor, placing your palm next to the inside arch of your front foot. For a deeper chest and shoulder opening, place your front hand on the outside of your front foot or on a yoga block.

Hold for up to 5 breaths.

To release, press firmly through your back foot. Then, exhale as you slowly come up to a standing position with your arms extended at shoulder height. Turn your feet and body so they face the same direction, then step your feet together. Return to the top of your mat and repeat on the opposite side.

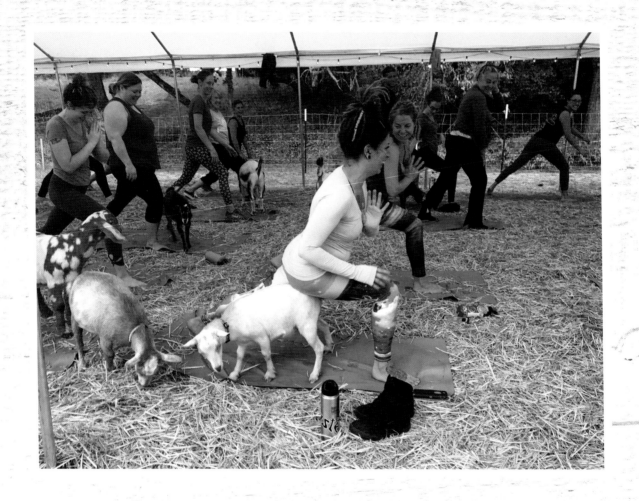

Hey, guys? How do I tell this nice lady that she's sitting on me without insulting her? Does she even know I'm here?

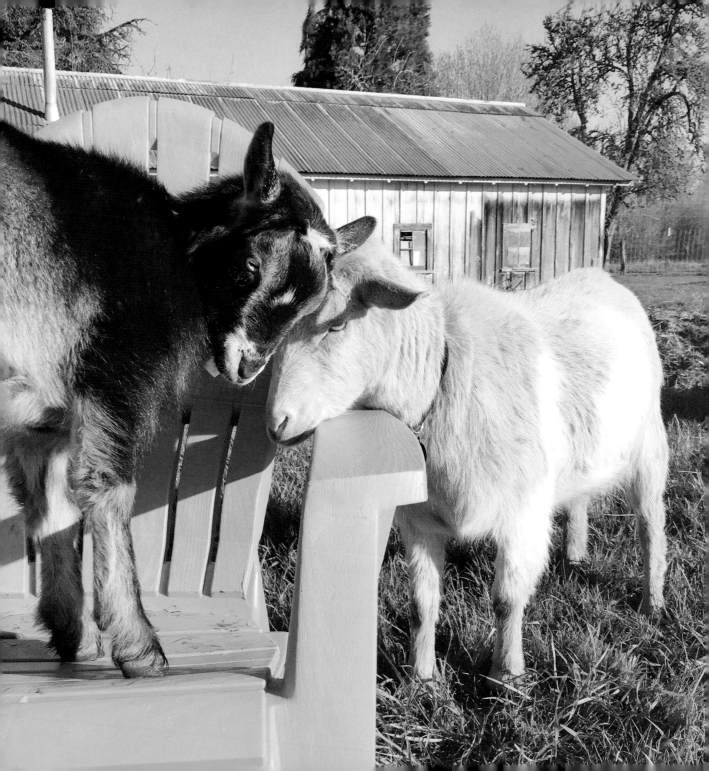

Child's Pose

BALASANA

From Table Top, exhale and lower your hips to your heels and your forehead to the floor. Have your knees together or, if more comfortable, spread your knees slightly apart.

Your arms can be overhead with your palms on the floor, bent with your palms or fists stacked under your forehead, or on the floor alongside your body with your palms up.

Breathe slowly and deeply, actively pressing your belly against your thighs on the inhale.

Breathe and hold for 4 to 12 breaths.

To release, place your palms under your shoulders and slowly inhale to a seated position.

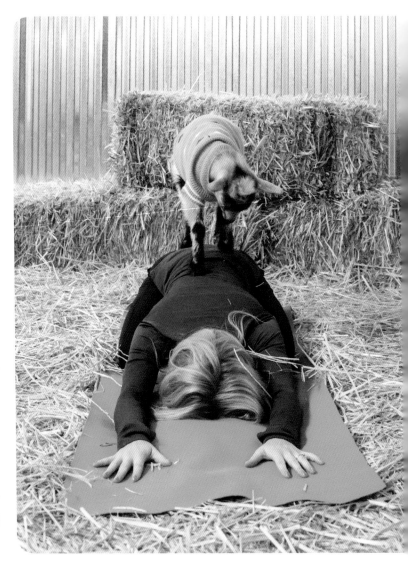

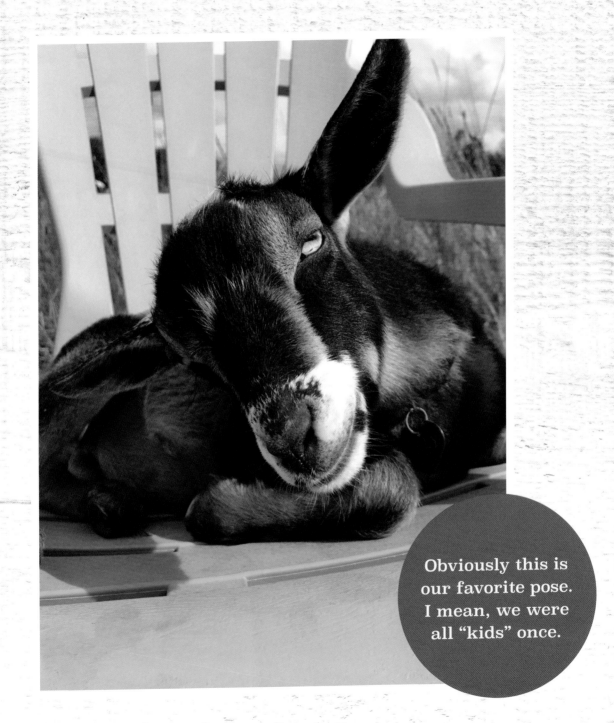

Obviously this is our favorite pose. I mean, we were all "kids" once.

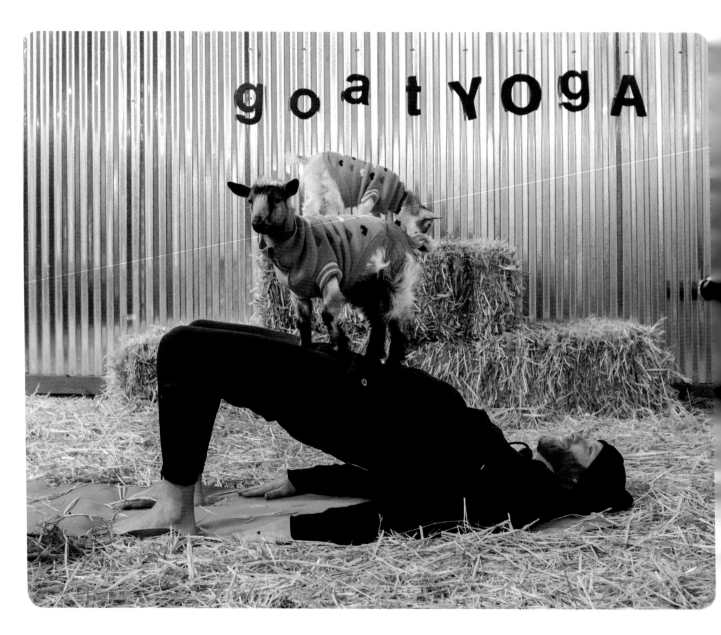

Bridge Pose

SETU BANDHA SARVANGASANA

Lie on your back with your knees bent and your feet on the floor. Extend your arms along the floor, palms flat.

Press your feet and arms firmly into the floor. Exhale as you lift your hips toward the ceiling.

Draw your tailbone toward your pubic bone, holding your buttocks off the floor. Do not squeeze your glutes or flex your buttocks.

Roll your shoulders back and underneath your body. Clasp your hands and extend your arms along the floor beneath your pelvis. Straighten your arms as much as possible, pressing your forearms into the mat. Reach your knuckles toward your heels.

Keep your thighs and feet parallel—do not roll to the outer edges of your feet or let your knees drop together. Press your weight evenly across all four corners of both feet. Lengthen your tailbone toward the backs of your knees.

Hold for up to 5 breaths. To release, unclasp your hands and place them palms down alongside your body. Exhale as you slowly roll your spine along the floor, vertebra by vertebra. Allow your knees to drop together.

restore

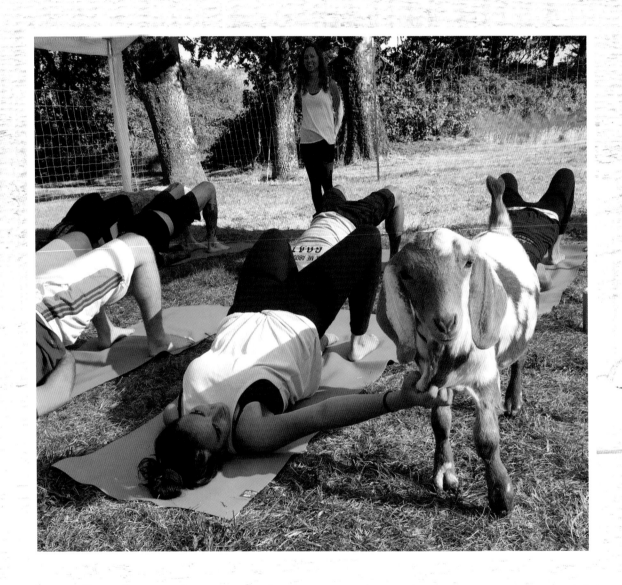

I'll tell you what I heard in class if you tell me.

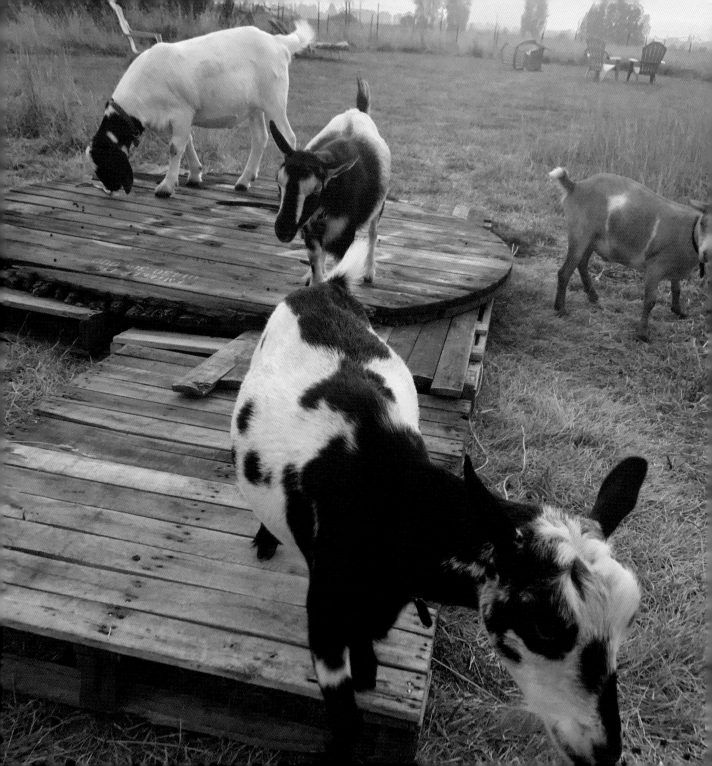

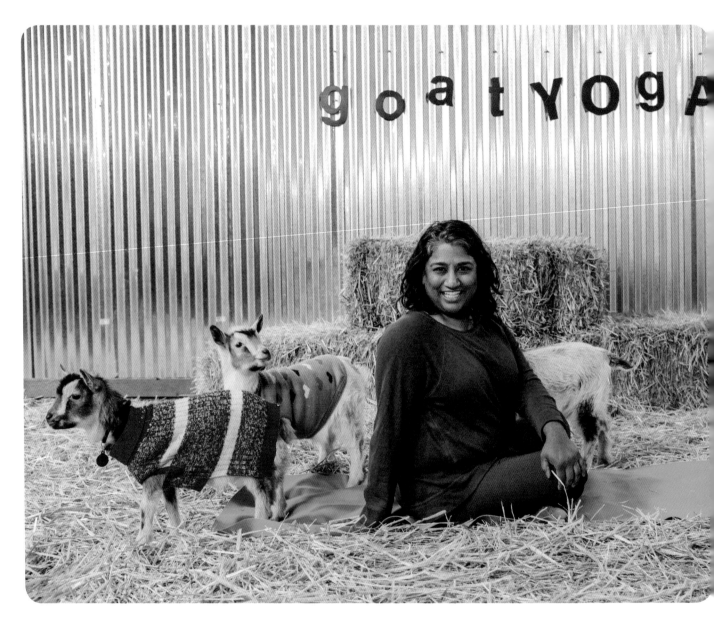

Seated Spinal Twist Pose

ARDHA MATSYENDRASANA

Sit on the edge of a firm blanket. Extend your legs in front of your body and sit up straight. Then, cross your legs in front of you at your shins. If your hips are very tight, you can sit on a bolster or block. With your knees wide, place each foot beneath the opposite knee. Fold your legs in toward your torso.

Balance your weight evenly across your sit bones. Align your head, neck, and spine. Lengthen your spine, but soften your neck. Relax your feet and thighs.

Place your right hand on the floor behind you. Bring your left hand to the outside of your right knee, exhaling as you gently twist to the right. Inhale again as you lengthen your spine, and exhale as you twist deeper. Gaze over your right shoulder. Do not push hard against your knee to force a deeper twist.

Keep your collarbone broad. Do not round your shoulders, and be sure to sit up straight. Do not lean your torso forward in order to obtain a deeper twist. Instead, twist only as far as you can go while keeping your head aligned directly over your tailbone.

Hold for up to 10 breaths.

Exhale as you come back to the center.

Change the cross of your legs and repeat the twist on the opposite side for the same length of time.

To release the pose, come back to the center.

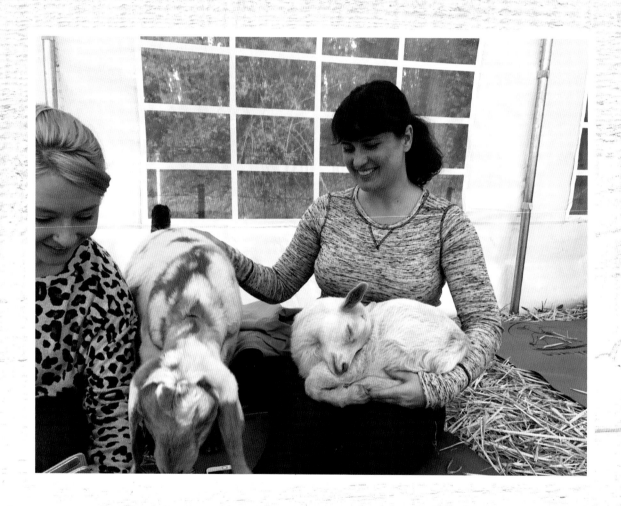

I'm meditating on what I will have to eat
once class is over.

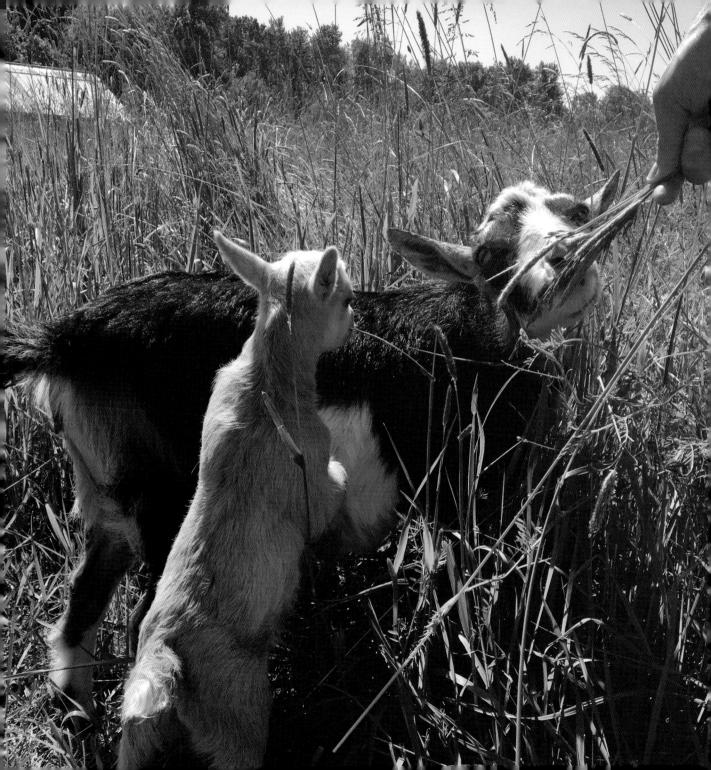

Bow Pose

DHANURASANA

Begin by lying flat on your stomach with your chin on the mat and your hands resting at your sides.

On an exhalation, bend your knees. Bring your heels as close as you can to your buttocks, keeping your knees hip-distance apart.

Reach back with both hands and hold on to your outer ankles.

On an inhale, lift your heels toward the ceiling, drawing your thighs up and off the mat. Your head, chest, and upper torso will also lift off the mat. Draw your tailbone down firmly into the floor while you simultaneously lift your heels and thighs even higher. Lift your chest and press your shoulder blades firmly into your upper back. Draw your shoulders away from your ears.

Gaze forward and breathe softly. Your breath will become shallow, but do not hold your breath.

Hold for up to 5 breaths.

To release, exhale and gently lower your thighs to the mat. Slowly release your legs and feet to the floor. Place your right ear on the mat, and relax your arms at your sides for a few breaths. Repeat the pose for the same amount of time, then rest with your left ear on the mat.

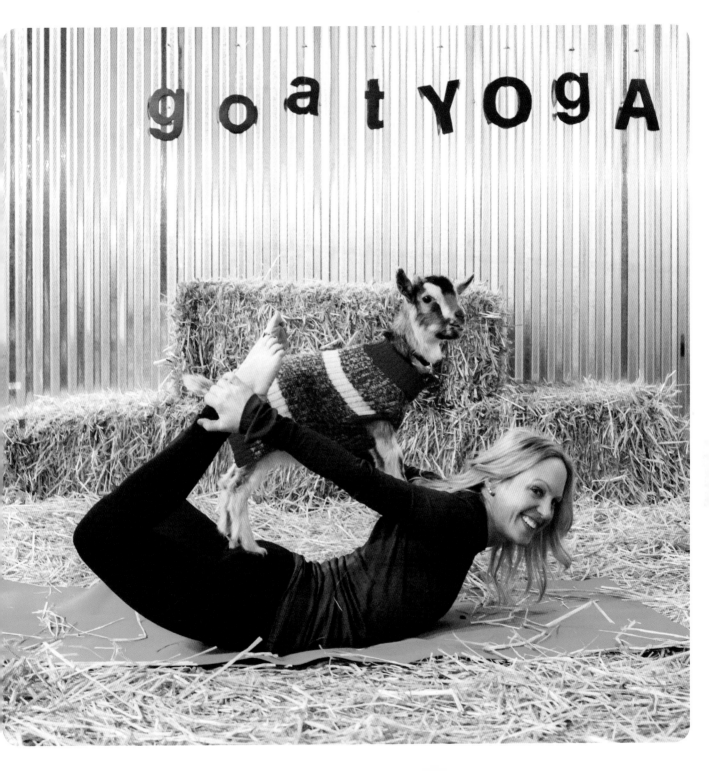

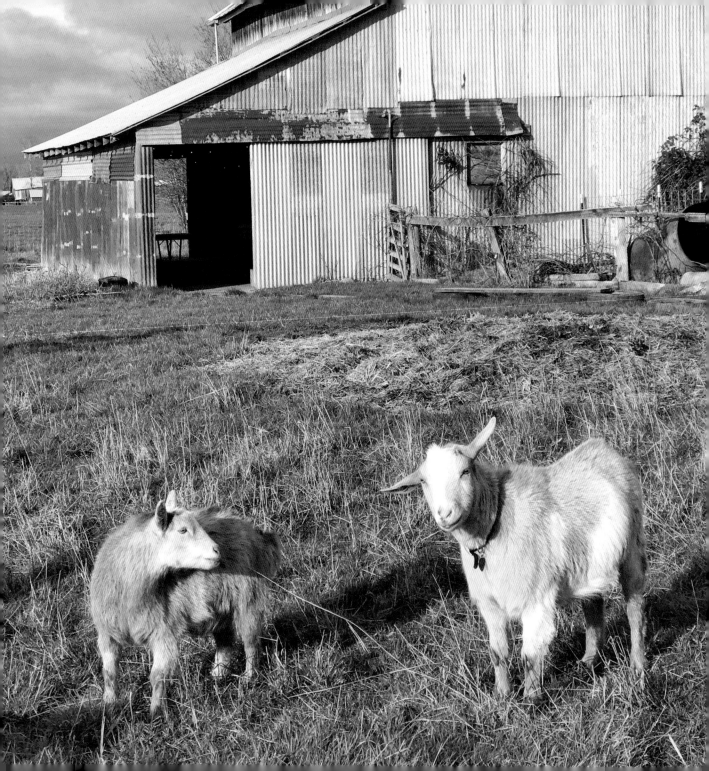

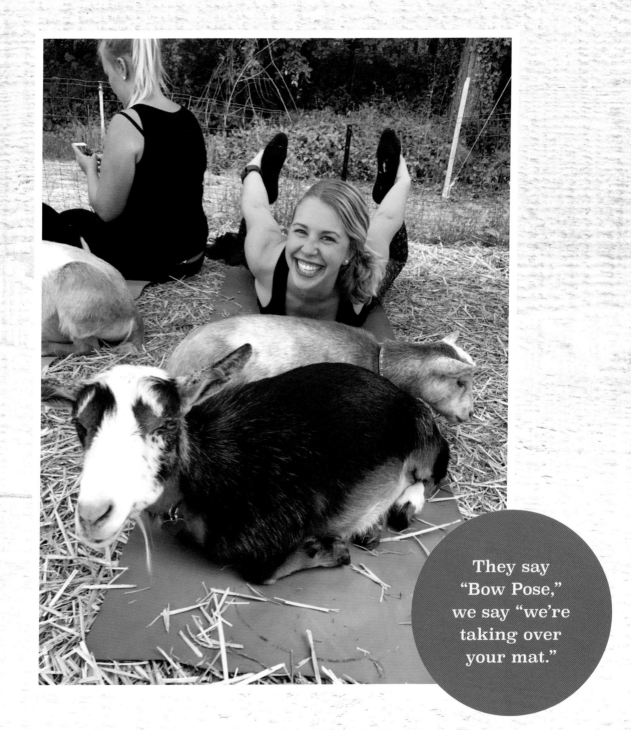

They say "Bow Pose," we say "we're taking over your mat."

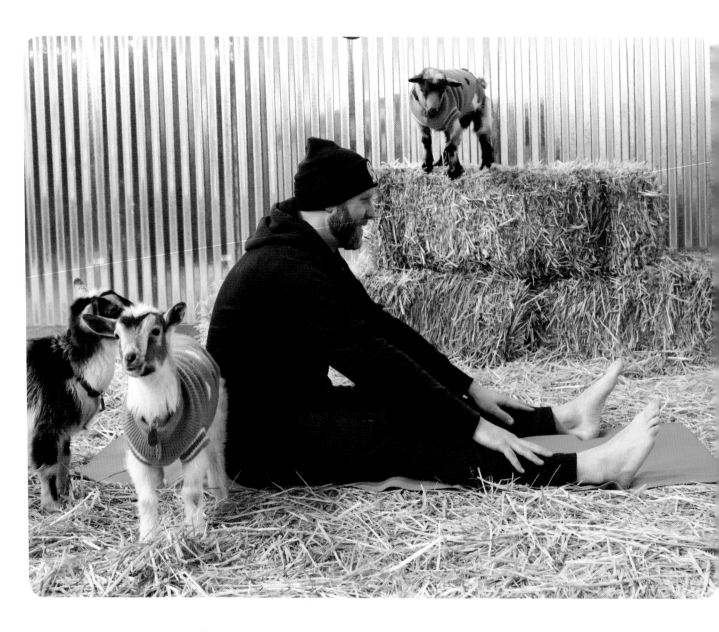

Seated Forward Bend Pose

PASCHIMOTTANASANA

Sit on the edge of a firm blanket with your legs extended in front of you. Reach actively through your heels. Beginners should bend their knees throughout the pose, eventually straightening their legs as flexibility increases.

Inhale as you reach your arms out to the side and then overhead, lengthening your spine.

Exhaling, bend forward from the hip joints. Do not bend at your waist. Lengthen the front of your torso. Imagine your torso coming to rest on your thighs instead of tipping your nose toward your knees.

Hold on to your shins, ankles, or feet—wherever your flexibility permits. You can also wrap a yoga strap or towel around the soles of your feet, holding it firmly with both hands.

Keep the front of your torso long; do not round your back. Let your belly touch your legs first and then your chest. Your head and nose should touch your legs last.

With each inhale, lengthen the front torso. With each exhale, fold a bit deeper.

Hold for up to 5 breaths. To release the pose, draw your tailbone toward the floor as you inhale and lift your torso.

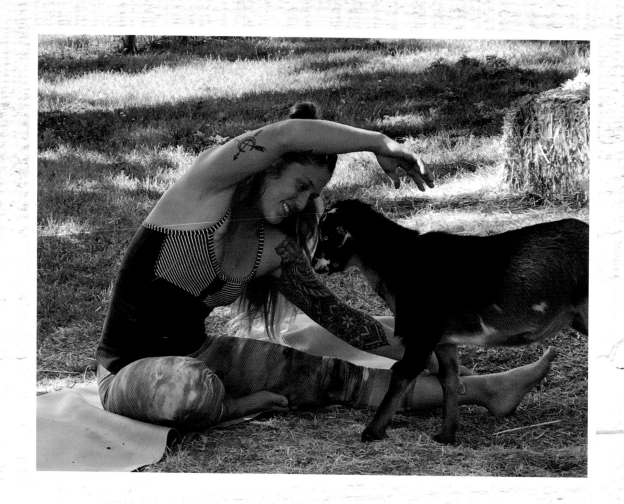

"Seated Forward Bend," or what I call
"an opportunity to pet me."

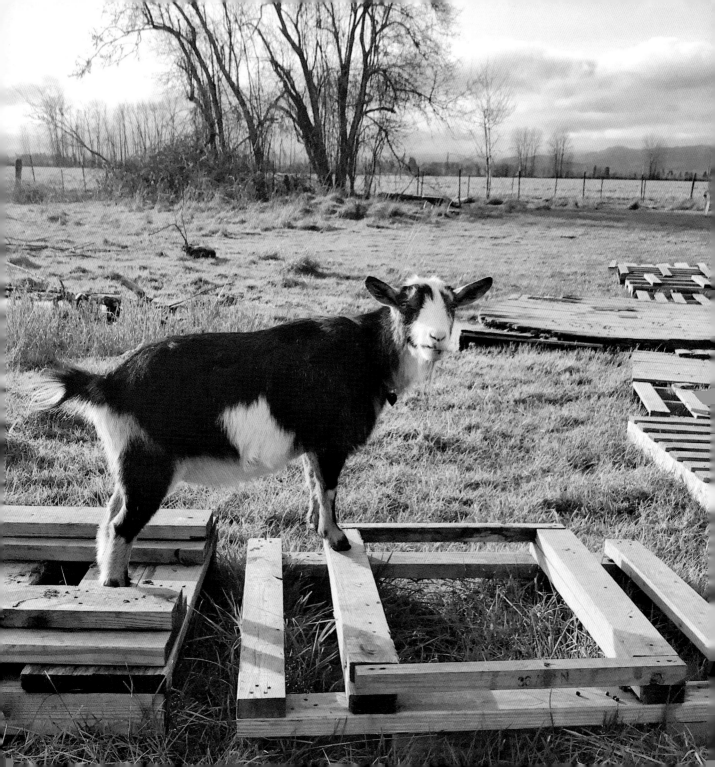

Final Relaxation

SAVASANA

Lying on your back, let your arms and legs drop open, with your arms about 45 degrees from the side of your body. Make sure you are warm and comfortable; if you need to, place blankets under or over your body.

Close your eyes, and take slow, deep breaths through your nose. Allow your whole body to become soft and heavy, letting it relax into the floor. As it relaxes, feel your whole body rising and falling with each breath.

Scan your body from your toes to your fingers to the crown of your head, looking for tension, tightness, and contracted muscles. Consciously release and relax any areas that you find. If you need to, rock or wiggle parts of your body from side to side to encourage further release.

Release all control of your breath, mind, and body. Let your body move deeper and deeper into a state of total relaxation.

Stay in *Savasana* for 5 to 15 minutes.

To release, slowly deepen your breath, wiggle your fingers and toes, reach your arms over your head, and stretch your whole body. Exhale while bending your knees into your chest, and roll over to one side, coming into a fetal position. When you are ready, slowly inhale up to a seated position.

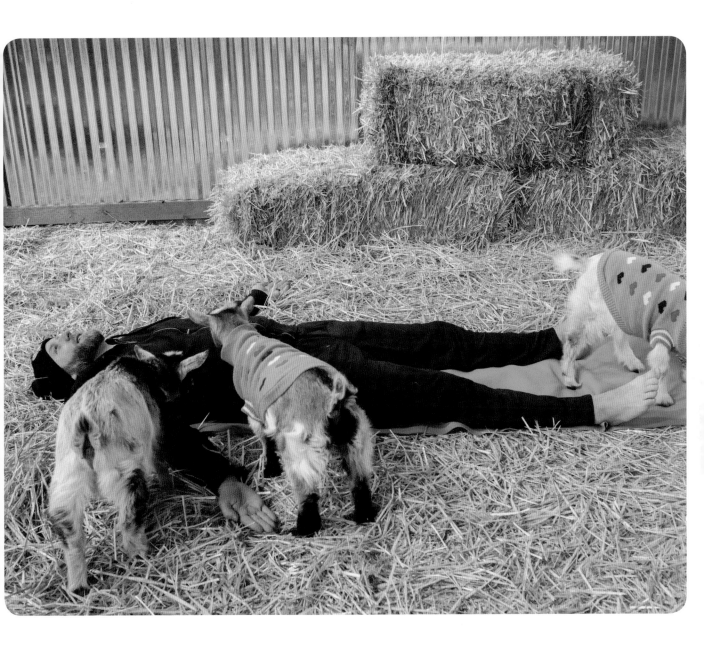

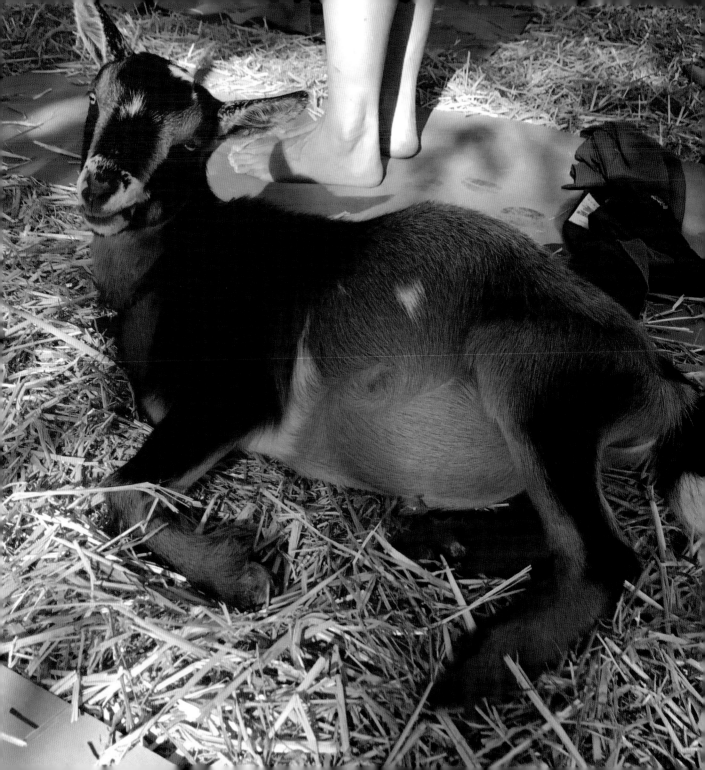

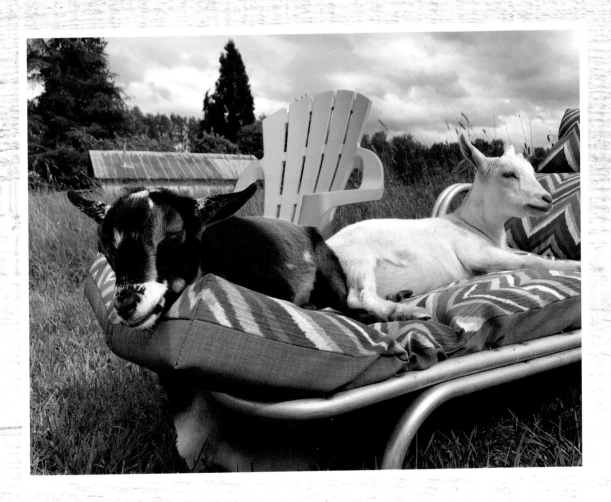

Usually we don't take anything lying down,
but we like to watch the humans release all of their stress.
We want them to goat away calm and relaxed.

ACKNOWLEDGMENTS

Sometimes, the simplest concept can change the world. Without the following people in my life, goat yoga would not be where it is today.

Heather Davis, the woman who inspired goat yoga: She is the most selfless, caring human on this planet. Without her, there would be far fewer happy people in the world.

My parents, Art and Ginny Morse: They have always been my biggest cheerleaders and my rocks. I'm so lucky to have them.

My daughter, Joslyn, and her family, who teach me every day that the most important things in life aren't money or things, but the memories we make together.

My boyfriend, Sean: This man has had to listen to me talk about all things goats for our entire relationship. I'm so thankful for his support every step of the way, being my rock, and most importantly loving me even when I'm a crazy anxiety monster.

My best friend, Jill: We share everything together and without her I'd be lost. She invests so much of her time helping me with strategies to help me succeed. She means the world to me.

My niece, Cielia, who is more like my soul sister: When I was recently diagnosed and not doing well, she—a single mom going through law school and at the busiest time of her life—still took the time to fly from Hawaii to Oregon to clean my barn, clean my house, and help me with the first goat yoga classes.

My friend Kristi, who believed in me enough to loan me money to get goat yoga off the ground and launch it into a legit business and more than just a little class in my back field. She is a rad human and I love her!

My friend Bronwyn: Goat yoga was going viral, I was so weak at times that I couldn't even feed myself. She would bring me groceries, check on me, and help me with classes. I'll never forget how wonderful she was to me and I love her.

Jackie Shaw, who is one of the most brilliant people I know. She has invested so much of her time and talent into helping me build this business. She is an avid animal lover and has been so dedicated from day one. I thank her for sharing her brilliant brain and warm heart with me.

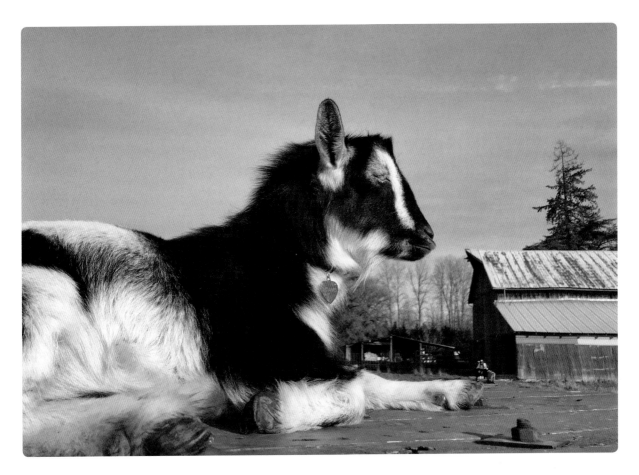

Alex Dyer, who will go down in history as the best ex-husband ever. He's one of my closest friends who has been there for me every step of the way and has gone above and beyond.

Kem: She has raised four baby goats in her house! She bottle fed throughout the night and changed diapers. This is not an easy task when you have twin baby goats jumping all over your house for a couple of months. She loved them and made sure that they were the most loving goat yoga goats on the planet.

Joan Demarest: She is the one that started my goat obsession by sharing Oscar and Peanut with me for a summer, before I knew I needed goats in my life. She changed my life with one act of kindness.

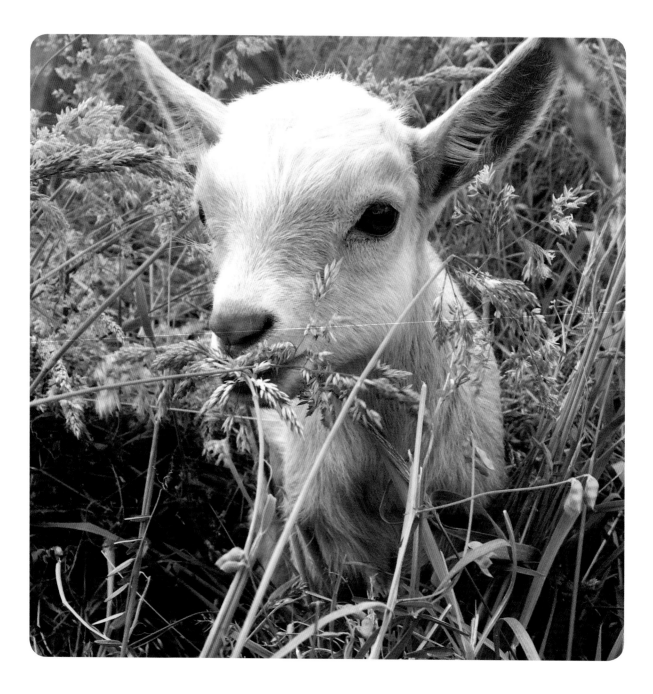

ABOUT THE AUTHOR

Originally from Michigan, Lainey Morse has lived in Oregon since 2006. Lainey has worked in the business development and marketing fields and is an award-winning professional photographer. She has a small hobby farm called No Regrets in the Willamette Valley where she lives with her 13 goats, four chickens, and three barn cats. She now works full-time on developing the Original Goat Yoga business.

Visit her and learn more at:

- goatyoga.net
- @goatyoga
- @GoatYogaOregon
- facebook.com/goatyoga

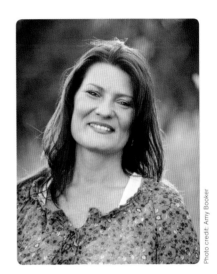

Photo credit: Amy Booker

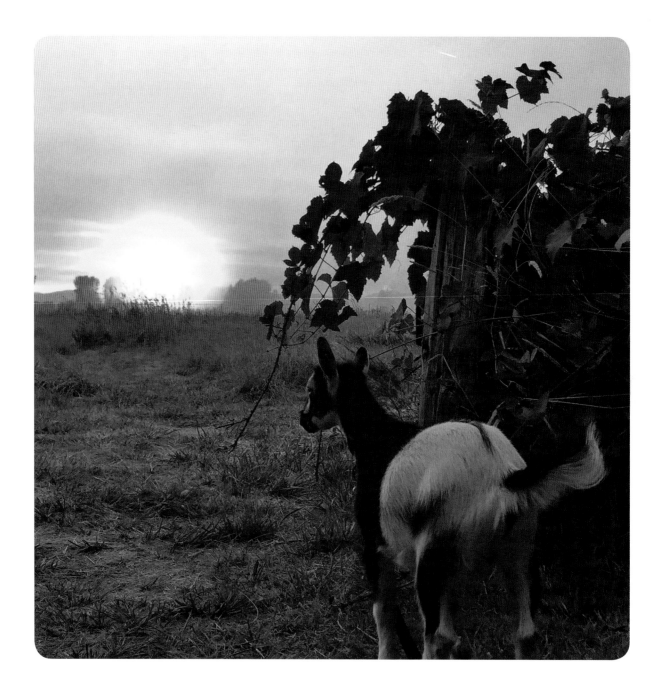